Pregnancy, Childbirth & Your Newborn Simplified

A Compact Handbook for Expectant Moms Covering Conception & Labor to Birthing & Beyond (Includes a Chapter on Healthy Recipes for Each Trimester!)

J.K. Karliese

This book belongs to :

YOUR FREE BONUS

Baby Health Tips

Common Infant Illnesses and How To Treat Them!

by JK Karliese

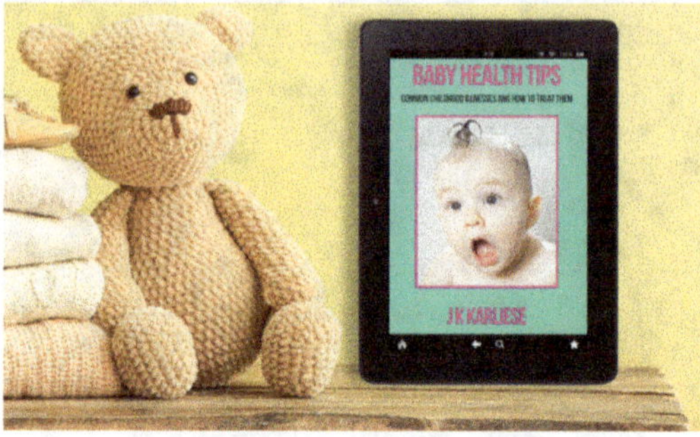

Worried about your newborn getting sick?

Inside this cheat sheet you'll:

- **Uncover & learn to identify the most common infant infections:** Even if you have no medical background!
- **Discover how to prevent and treat the most common infant infections:** Learn EXACTLY what to do to prevent infections and to minimize symptoms (if already present). Learn how to begin helping your baby before you get to the doctor's office!
- **Build up your confidence as a new mom:** Gain the necessary knowledge to build up your confidence in your ability to properly care for your baby!

Tell us where to send your free bonus!

Please send me the bonus! Click here

http://subscribepage.io/Karliese-Baby-Health-Tips

or Scan QR code

To All Moms, Moms-To-Be, and Aspiring Moms-To-Be:

You are each unique in your journey to motherhood, yet bound to each other by a shared inner strength that cannot fully be explained. My hope is for this book to empower and lead you through an exciting adventure to many more self-discoveries.

Contents

Behold, children are a heritage from the Lord, the fruit of the womb is a reward – Psalm 127:3 (NKJV)

Introduction

You've been dreaming about this moment your entire life, and now it's finally here—the best news you could ever hope to receive! Perhaps you can still hear the doctor's words as they handed you the lab report: "You are pregnant." Or maybe you discovered it on your own using a home pregnancy kit, with two undeniably visible solid lines in the testing well. Regardless of how you found out, you're likely flooded with a whirlwind of emotions: shock, joy, excitement, fear, anticipation, and more.

While the journey to this point might differ for each woman, most would agree that it's an incredibly special and unforgettable moment in their lives. Embarking on the pregnancy journey marks an exceptional period in a woman's life, involving profound changes that unfold over nine miraculous months. Amid the uncertainties that lie ahead, there are also precious moments to cherish. Your story is unique and deserving of the best guidance and support possible. That's where this book comes in: *Pregnancy, Childbirth & Your Newborn*. It is here to meet those needs by providing the answers you seek and the guidance and support you require.

You may be reading this as a new mom-to-be experiencing your first pregnancy. Please know that it's okay to feel anxious in your journey, perhaps even overwhelmed, but rest assured that the *Pregnancy, Childbirth & Your Newborn* handbook is specifically crafted to provide the knowledge you need to boost your confidence throughout this experience.

My name is J.K. Karliese, and I proudly embrace two roles that appear to be worlds apart but are linked by a common thread of compassion and knowledge. I take this stage as an independent writer and book publisher. But beneath this professional identity lies a more personal one: an experienced bedside nurse and an advanced practice nurse professional with a passion for health education, advocacy, and counseling, focusing mainly on women and children.

I've been in the nursing profession for over nine years, working in family practice, pediatrics, and cardiology. I've witnessed life's miraculous stories, held hands during uncertain times, and shared the successes and tribulations of countless people, including women like yourself. It was in these moments that I discovered my calling and a strong need to convert my skills into relatable ways that would appeal to a larger audience, including individuals such as yourself.

Also, as a mother of two young children, I am very attuned to the heartbeat of my readers—both first-time and experienced mothers who find themselves navigating pregnancy's uncharted waters. I understand their hopes, concerns, anxieties, fears, and curiosity. I've walked the path of motherhood and have also been the one to provide care, guidance, and support to others on the same path.

I wish to leave a reassuring and guiding impact on the minds of expectant mothers (both young and mature). I want to be the voice that comforts amidst doubt, the light that illuminates the route ahead. I hope to bridge the gap between the known and the unknown in the pages of *Pregnancy, Childbirth & Your Newborn* by offering explanations, insights, and solace along the road.

And why pick this book from among the many options available to you? As you read this book, you will gain access to expert advice on prenatal care, decode the labor process, and learn how to embrace the wonderful chaos that is postpartum life. This book will also help you separate the facts from the myths regarding the pregnancy journey.

You might be wondering why the focus of this guide is on first-time mothers. The reason is simple: This book addresses each stage of the journey in a simple, easy-to-understand language, without being condescending and treating you like a child on the one hand or overwhelming you with medical jargon on the other. It seeks to empower you with informed decisions every step of the way. This book is envisioned as a reliable guide and an unwavering fountain of knowledge that goes beyond just being informational. It is filled with reservoirs of knowledge and insights and packaged as a non-bulky, purse-and-pocket-friendly, daily companion.

It is worth mentioning that embracing motherhood at a more mature age is a blessing, and I will highlight the benefits and joys that come with this experience. From the depth of emotional readiness to the pile of life experiences you bring as a mature mom-to-be, there's a richness to this journey that is simply astounding. But beyond the practicalities, I will also look at the emotional and psychological components of becoming a parent and also the evolution of your own identity.

So, whether you're taking this path after saying your vows as a newlywed or you are a single professional woman with or without a partner, this pregnancy guide stands by your side as you eagerly anticipate the pitter-patter of little feet. It's an ally for newlyweds, unwed couples, and single moms. With its gentle guidance, you can navigate the complexities of pregnancy, prepare for your baby's arrival, and confidently enter motherhood.

Undoubtedly, knowledge has the power to illuminate the unknown. With *Pregnancy, Childbirth & Your Newborn*, you will be capable of making decisions that align with your unique situation, thereby crafting a personalized journey. Apart from covering every aspect of pregnancy, labor, and childbirth, I have included a bonus chapter that outlines the components of one full day of nutritious meal plans for each trimester. This will help ensure that you are nourishing yourself and your precious bundle in the healthiest possible way.

Finally, as you dive into the pages that follow, remember this: You are not alone. You are part of an extraordinary lineage of mothers who have taken this path before you. Every step in your journey is a testament to the strength and resilience that lies within you. Through this book, I want you to envision me as your ally, walking alongside you, ensuring your journey is one marked by knowledge, power, and the joy of nurturing new life. Come, let's embark on this adventure together, turning the pages of learning, discovery, and anticipation, and being united by the common thread that binds us all: motherhood.

Part One

Preconception Care – Planning Your Pregnancy

Making the decision to have a child is momentous. It is to decide forever to have your heart go walking around outside your body.

— Elizabeth Stone

If you don't know your options, you don't have any.

— Diana Korte

Chapter 1

Understanding the concepts of Fertility, Conception, and Optimized Conception

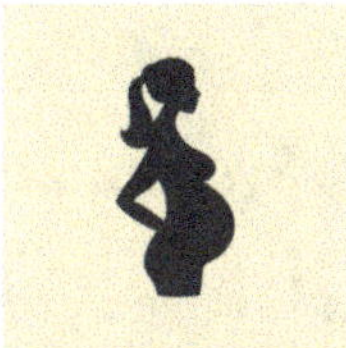

This chapter aims to introduce some key concepts, discuss how the human body (male and female) works when it comes to having babies, and touch on potential ways to improve the chances of getting pregnant.

1.1: Concepts: Understanding the Reproductive System and the Concept of Fertility

The human reproductive system is a complex yet well-coordinated organ system designed to create an environment conducive to generating and sustaining a new life that eventually results in the birth of a baby.

The concept of fertility is central to this system. It refers to how capable a woman's body is of becoming pregnant and having a child. Fertility depends on a complex balance of hormones and organs, such as the ovaries, which produce eggs, and the uterus, which carries and nurtures the fertilized egg into a full-term baby.

The Reproductive Journey: A Story of Two Genders

This amazing journey of reproduction comprises two pivotal players: the male and female reproductive systems. Each system, distinct in its own right, comes together in a symphony of biology leading to the production of new life. It is a story about nurturing, growth, and the harmonious union of two halves into a whole.

The Male Reproductive System: Life's Building Blocks

Consider the male reproductive system to be a factory that manufactures the building components of life. It revolves around the testes, where sperm—the microscopic agents of fertilization—are painstakingly manufactured. These small, tadpole-like cells are fostered, grown, and prepared for their epic journey through a process known as *spermatogenesis*.

These sperm are propelled through the vas deferens (sperm duct) by ejaculation, which acts as a launchpad for their voyage. What is their final destination? The female reproductive system, where the sperms embark on a quest to mate with an egg, sets in motion the spectacular adventure of conception.

Male Reproductive System

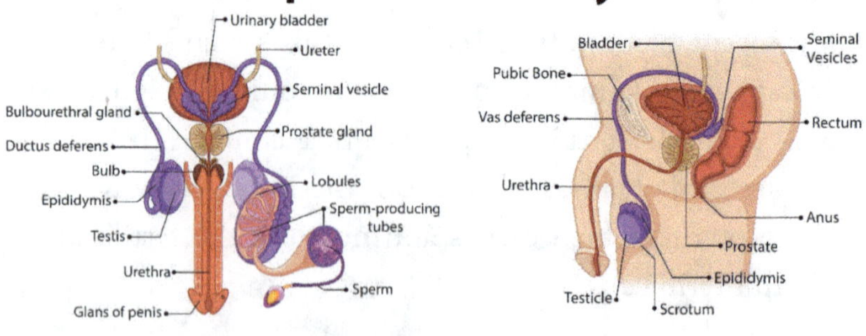

The Female Reproductive System: Sustaining the Miracle

In parallel, the female reproductive system provides a nurturing refuge for potential life. The ovaries may be compared to nature's treasure chests because they contain thousands of potential eggs. Every month, one egg is chosen for ovulation and begins its journey down the fallopian tube.

If a sperm successfully meets an egg during this journey, a remarkable transformation takes place: fertilization, the merger of two separate entities into a zygote. This tiny zygote travels to the uterine lining, where it nestles in preparation for the chance of developing into a baby.

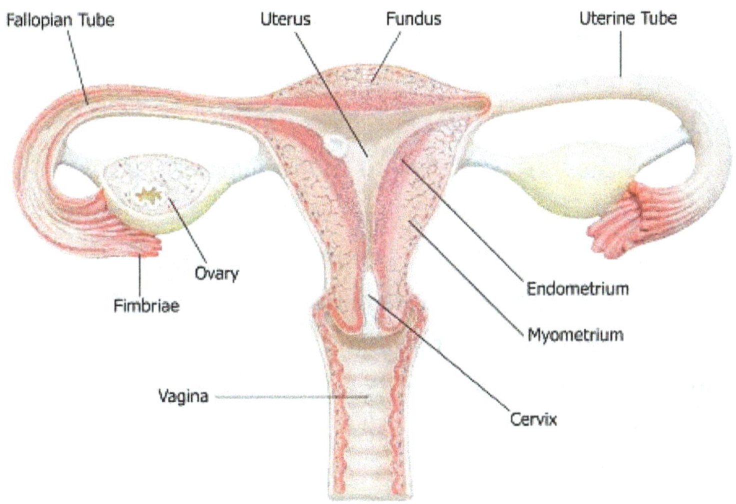

Female Reproductive System

The uterus is the nurturing haven that provides the ideal environment for the zygote to embed and grow from an immature embryo into a fully mature fetus that is ready to be born after the nine-month gestation period. If fertilization does not occur, the uterine lining is shed through menstruation, signaling the end of one chapter and the start of a new cycle of possibilities.

1.2: Tips for Optimizing Your Chances of Conceiving

Knowing your body's natural cycles, particularly the process of ovulation, is essential for improving your chances of conception. Here's a list of tips to help you make informed decisions and increase your chances of conceiving successfully.

- **Understanding ovulation:** Ovulation is the pivotal moment in your menstrual cycle when an egg is released from the ovary, allowing for fertilization.
- **Tracking your cycle:** For a few months, carefully record the start date of your menstrual periods and monitor your basal body temperature. This baseline data can help you predict your fertile days.
- **Observing ovulation signs:** Keep an eye out for changes in the consistency and texture of cervical mucus, as well as any mild abdominal discomfort, which indicates that ovulation is near. Cervical mucus during ovulation is clear, egg-white-like, with a stretchy consistency that facilitates sperm motility.
- **Ovulation prediction kits:** These may be purchased without a prescription and can be used to detect hormonal surges preceding ovulation through a simple urine test.

- **Calculating your fertile window:** You can estimate the range of days during which conception is most likely to occur by subtracting approximately 14 days from the whole duration of your monthly cycle.
- **Regular intimacy:** Maintain a constant schedule of sexual activity throughout your reproductive window, keeping in mind that sperm can dwell inside the female body for several days (Marcin, 2017).
- **Prioritizing a healthy lifestyle:** Maintain a healthy diet, engage in regular physical activity, properly handle stress, and avoid dangerous behaviors such as smoking and excessive alcohol intake.
- **Seeking professional guidance:** If conception remains elusive after several months of attempting, consult with a healthcare professional who can provide personalized insights and suggest potential strategies.

1.3: Prioritizing Preconception Care

Before embarking on the journey to conception, it is crucial to place a strong emphasis on preconception care. Consulting with your women's health provider is an essential step in this process. This healthcare professional is qualified to take you through the intricacies of preparing for pregnancy. Your choice of a women's health provider depends on your needs and comfort.

In the United States, you have the option of choosing from the following: a medically trained obstetrician (MD), an advanced practice registered nurse midwife, or a licensed physician assistant working under the guidance of an MD. For the actual birthing process, some women have shown a preference for unorthodox naturalistic birth plans and, therefore, employ the services of a doula. None of these choices is wrong; it all depends on each individual's preference.

Preconception care often involves dealing with any underlying medical conditions before getting pregnant. Some of these conditions are

- diabetes
- hypertension
- congenital heart issues
- blood diseases like sickle cell anemia

Addressing these and other disorders that might have an impact on pregnancy is vital. Timely diagnosis and treatment of these conditions not only enhance your overall health but also have a substantial effect on the well-being of both you and your future child. Your women's health provider will play a vital role in ensuring that your preconception journey is well-informed, well-prepared, and optimized for a successful pregnancy.

1.4: Preconception Nutrition and Supplementation

Proper Nutrition in Pregnancy: What Is a Healthy Balanced Diet for a Pregnant Woman?

A healthy, balanced diet for a pregnant woman is all about giving the correct mix of nutrients that support the well-being of both the mother and her growing baby. It comprises a mix of meals that provide vital vitamins, minerals, and proteins, while also avoiding foods that might pose risks during pregnancy. This balanced approach ensures a strong foundation for a smooth and healthy pregnancy journey.

Here are some important guidelines for preconception nutrition and safe food choices during pregnancy.

Foods to Eat

- **Foods high in folate:** Leafy greens, beans, lentils, and fortified cereals are high in folate, a B vitamin important for preventing birth abnormalities in the baby's spine and brain.
- **Iron-rich foods:** Lean meats, legumes, and whole grains contain the iron required to prevent anemia and sustain the increased blood volume during pregnancy.
- **Calcium sources:** Dairy products, fortified plant-based milk, and leafy greens provide the calcium required for strong bones and teeth in both you and your baby.
- **Omega-3 fatty acids:** Include fatty fish (low in mercury), chia seeds, and walnuts for brain and vision development in the baby.

Foods to Avoid: What You Should *Not* Eat While Pregnant

Certain foods can be hazardous to your health and the health of your growing baby. Safeguarding your pregnancy means avoiding potential dangers.

- **Mercury-rich seafood:** While fish is an excellent source of Omega-3s, avoid high-mercury seafood such as shark, swordfish, king mackerel, and tilefish. Choose low-mercury options such as salmon, shrimp, and cod.
- **Unpasteurized dairy products:** Listeria monocytogenes, a dangerous bacterium, can lurk in unpasteurized dairy products, increasing the risk of illness. To be safe, stick to pasteurized varieties.
- **Raw or undercooked seafood:** Sushi and raw shellfish can expose you to harmful bacteria and parasites. Choose cooked alternatives to reduce potential risks.
- **Contaminated seafood and unwashed produce:** Contaminated seafood and unwashed fruits and vegetables can harbor germs such as E. coli, salmonella, shigella, and others, which can cause gastrointestinal infection. Proper cooking and thorough washing help to reduce these risks.
- **Undercooked eggs, poultry, and meats:** Undercooked eggs, poultry, and meats can harbor harmful bacteria like salmonella. Ensuring these foods are cooked to the recommended temperatures is essential to avoid foodborne diseases during pregnancy.

Guidelines for Preparing Food During Pregnancy

When preparing food for a pregnant woman, it's important to prioritize hygiene to look after her health and that of the growing baby. Here are some guidelines to follow:

- **Clean hands and surfaces:** Before dealing with any food items, thoroughly cleanse your hands using soap and water. Additionally, make certain that all utensils, cutting boards, and surfaces are clean and sanitized.
- **Separate raw ingredients from prepared dishes:** Cross-contamination can be prevented by keeping raw meats, poultry, seafood, and eggs separate from ready-to-eat foods. Ensure you have separate cutting boards and utensils for handling raw and cooked foods.
- **Safe cooking temperatures:** Cook meat, poultry, seafood, and eggs to their recommended safe internal temperatures. A food thermometer can assist in ensuring that they're fully cooked and clear of harmful bacteria.
- **Proper refrigeration:** Refrigerate perishable foods right away and keep your refrigerator at a safe temperature (below 40°F or 4°C). This stops bacteria from rapidly multiplying.

1.5: Weight Gain During Pregnancy

When it comes to gaining weight during pregnancy, finding that sweet spot is necessary for both you and your baby's well-being. Here's all you need to know about what's too much, too little, and whether you really need to eat for two.

Finding the Right Balance

- **Too much weight gain:** While some additional weight is normal during pregnancy, gaining too much might increase the risk of problems such as gestational diabetes and high blood pressure. To stay on track, aim for modest weight gain within the recommended range.

- **Too little weight gain:** Inadequate weight gain can also cause problems, resulting in a baby with low birth weight. Finding the right balance ensures your baby receives the nourishment they need for healthy growth.

Eating for Two: Quality Over Quantity

Contrary to popular belief, you do not need to eat for two full-grown adults. Your baby's needs are a lot smaller than you might think. Instead of piling on more servings, focus on the quality of your meals. Select nutrient-dense foods that have the vitamins and minerals needed for your baby to develop properly.

Portion Control: Listening to Your Body

While there's no one-size-fits-all solution to portion sizes, It's important to pay attention to your body's hunger and fullness cues. Smaller, more frequent meals can aid digestion and alleviate nausea. Pregnancy weight gain is determined by individual factors such as starting weight and activity level, with healthcare providers offering personalized advice based on specific circumstances.

A well-balanced diet is recommended for both maternal and fetal health. Furthermore, the next chapter will discuss potential vices that may have an impact on the delicate process of conception and pregnancy, emphasizing the importance of caution and awareness for the health of both mother and child.

Chapter 2

The Vices—TACOS, Teratogens, and Treatment Medications

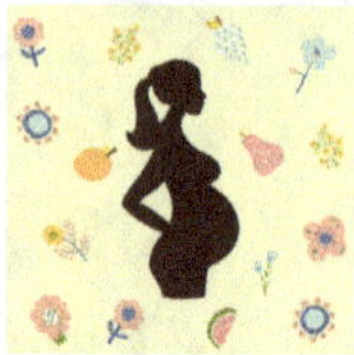

2.1: TACOS: What Are They?

The vices of pregnancy are factors that may result in negative outcomes in pregnancy. These vices include a range of harmful elements that can impact both the expectant mother's health and the growth of her baby. The acronym TACOS represents the five major vices of pregnancy: Tobacco, Alcohol, Caffeine, Opioids, and Stress. Each of these vices significantly affects pregnancy in today's modern world. These will be examined more closely in the following segments.

Tobacco (Smoking)

Tobacco, a plant product with a centuries-old history, has grave consequences, especially when combined with the pregnancy journey. Among the different methods of consumption, smoking is the most common. However, its seemingly harmless smoke causes dual detrimental effects, casting a shadow not only on the expectant mother but also on the delicate life she carries within her.

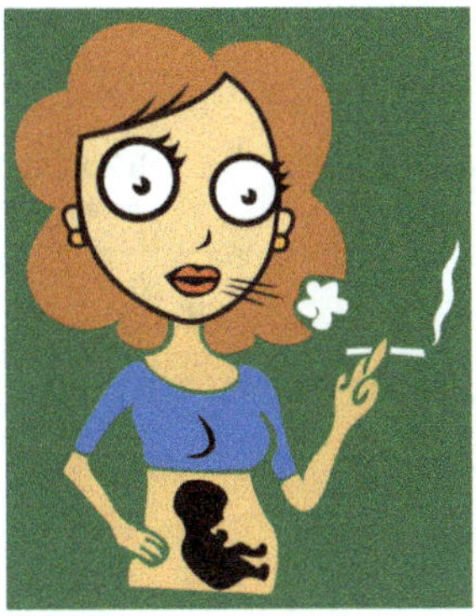

Harmful Effects: Smoking Versus Secondhand Smoke Exposure

Smoking is like a harmful fog that lingers over an unborn child. When a pregnant woman smokes, harmful substances such as nicotine, carbon monoxide, tar, benzene, and tobacco-specific nitrosamines enter the mother's bloodstream by simple diffusion and, from there, are transported to the baby during the transplacental blood exchange between the mother and the fetus. These agents constitute a deadly combination that can cause major issues, influencing not only the baby's growth but also raising the likelihood of birth defects and pregnancy complications.

But what if you're not the one smoking? Secondhand smoke, the unwelcome guest in this situation, is just as harmful. Breathing in the fumes generated by another person's cigarette can still expose your baby to these harmful substances, raising the risk of low birth weight, premature delivery, and developmental issues.

Alcohol

Unlike some lifestyle choices with a possible gray area, the verdict on alcohol is clear: There is no safe amount of alcohol during pregnancy (NIAAA, 2022). When a pregnant woman drinks, the alcohol travels in the bloodstream to the unborn baby through the placenta. Because the baby's developing organs, including the liver, do not have the capacity to process alcohol in the same way as an adult's organs, even a small amount of alcohol can be extremely toxic to the baby with harmful consequences.

Caffeine

The aroma of morning coffee is a ritual for many people, but during pregnancy, finding the appropriate caffeine balance becomes imperative. While caffeine can provide a nice energy boost, it is crucial to limit intake. The good news is that caffeine does not need to be taken off the table completely. Most experts agree that moderate caffeine usage (approximately 200 milligrams per day, or the equivalent of a 12-ounce cup of coffee) is safe for most pregnant women (Meixner, 2018). However, it is worth noting that caffeine is not limited to morning coffee; it is also found in tea, sodas, and even chocolate.

Opioids (and Other Narcotics)

For pregnant women who are battling opioid addiction, getting medical help is of the utmost importance. Nonetheless, discontinuing opiate usage suddenly can lead to withdrawal symptoms, posing potential risks to both the mother and her infant. Healthcare experts can give advice on adopting a safe approach that may include medications to help manage withdrawal while lowering risks to the baby. Premature birth, low birth weight, and other problems can result from opioid usage during pregnancy. Furthermore, research highlights that opioids can travel via the placenta to the newborn, potentially producing Neonatal Abstinence Syndrome (NAS), in which the baby experiences withdrawal after birth (NIH, 2020).

Stress

Pregnancy is a transformative period, full of anticipation and excitement, but it can also come with its share of stressors. Navigating the physical and emotional changes that come with bearing a life can be difficult. Moreover, stress isn't just about feeling overwhelmed—it can have real physiological effects on both the mother and her developing baby. When stress becomes chronic, it can cause the release of stress hormones, thereby altering blood flow to the uterus and impacting fetal growth. In addition, a woman's emotional state can resonate with her baby, potentially influencing their emotional development.

2.2: Other Vices to Avoid

Marijuana (Cannabis)

As societal views on marijuana change, its impact on pregnancy remains a concern. THC (delta-9-tetrahydrocannabinol), the main ingredient in cannabis, can get past the placental barrier and potentially impact embryonic development. According to research, prenatal THC exposure may cause problems with children's attention, memory, and cognitive function (CDC, 2020). If you're thinking about getting pregnant, talk to your doctor about your marijuana use for guidance.

2.3: What Are Teratogens?

Teratogens are chemicals or factors that can disrupt normal fetal development. These comprise various medications, chemicals, and diseases. Their potential to cause birth abnormalities or developmental issues emphasizes the need to be cautious during pregnancy. Furthermore, teratogens strike during the key phases of embryonic development when organs and systems are developing. They can produce a variety of problems, ranging from structural abnormalities to cognitive deficits.

2.4: Effects of TACOS and Teratogens on Pregnancy

Read on to learn about some of the most serious consequences of teratogen exposure during pregnancy, focusing on the effects of teratogens on fetal development and probable pregnancy outcomes.

- **Fetal alcohol syndrome (FAS):** Consuming alcohol during pregnancy can cause FAS, resulting in facial abnormalities, developmental disorders, and learning difficulties in the baby.
- **Low birth weight:** Babies may be born with a lower weight than estimated, which can cause health issues and a longer road to growth and development.
- **Intrauterine growth restriction:** Teratogens could hinder the baby's growth within the womb, resulting in intrauterine growth restriction. This can result in

smaller-than-expected newborns with potential health concerns.
- **Placental abruption:** The risk of placental abruption can be enhanced because of teratogens. This is a dangerous disorder in which the placenta prematurely detaches from the uterine wall, causing bleeding and endangering both the mother and her baby.
- **Placenta previa:** Teratogens may contribute to placenta previa, a condition in which the placenta partially or completely covers the cervix. This condition can cause bleeding and complications during pregnancy.
- **Miscarriage and stillbirth:** Teratogen exposure increases the chance of miscarriage (loss of the pregnancy before 20 weeks) and stillbirth (loss of the baby after 20 weeks). These are emotionally difficult experiences for expectant parents.
- **Premature labor:** Preterm labor can be triggered, resulting in contractions and the cervix opening before the baby is ready for birth. Premature babies might face health challenges because of their underdeveloped systems.

2.5: Infectious Teratogenic Organisms

The threat posed by infectious teratogenic organisms is an often overlooked aspect. These microscopic organisms can have a substantial impact on the course of a pregnancy, potentially leading to a variety of issues. Here are the details:

- **Cytomegalovirus (CMV):** Although this common virus may not cause symptoms in adults, it can harm the baby if contracted during pregnancy. It can cause hearing or visual issues, intellectual difficulties, and even miscarriage.
- **Toxoplasmosis:** Toxoplasma gondii, a parasite found in cat feces, can be dangerous. While this fluffy pet is adorable, it is crucial to avoid handling cat litter while pregnant to prevent exposure to this dangerous parasite, which can cause major problems in the baby's eyes, brain, or other organs.
- **Rubella (German measles):** Rubella can cause birth abnormalities or miscarriages in a developing baby. It is crucial to ensure you are immune through vaccination before pregnancy.
- **Varicella (chickenpox):** Contracting chickenpox while pregnant can be dangerous for both mother and child. Avoiding exposure is vital for pregnant women who have not had chickenpox or the vaccine.
- **Herpes simplex:** Having a genital herpes outbreak close to the due date, puts the baby at risk of contracting it during delivery. A healthcare practitioner can offer advice on how to handle this.
- **Chlamydia:** While it seldom causes birth abnormalities, untreated chlamydia can result in premature birth or low birth weight. Prenatal care and screenings are essential.

2.6: Some Less Common but Important Environmental Chemical Teratogens

While it's not always feasible to avoid every exposure, being knowledgeable helps you make informed choices. Remember, the path to parenthood is about embracing the wonders and challenges and protecting your baby from possible risks is just one of the many ways you are already excelling as a parent-to-be.

Our surroundings have lesser-known but pertinent environmental toxins that can impact a developing baby. Some of these include

- **Mercury compounds:** Found in some fish, mercury compounds can have a harmful impact on the baby's nervous system and brain development. Buy seafood low in mercury and avoid high-exposure areas. Women should be aware that certain beauty products, such as skin bleaching creams/lotions and soaps, contain mercury compounds and, therefore, are not advised for use during pregnancy. It is always a good idea to be familiar with the components of your beauty regimen.
- **Polychlorinated biphenyl (PCB):** These chemicals, commonly found in contaminated water or old electrical equipment, can endanger your baby's growth and development. Avoid exposure and be cautious around potential sources.
- **Herbicides:** Beautifying a yard or garden might involve herbicides, but these chemicals can harbor potential risks for pregnancy. Reduce exposure by

using alternative methods or hiring the services of a professional gardener.

- **Industrial solvents:** Exposure to industrial solvents in certain work environments or through contaminated air or water can have serious implications for a developing baby. It's important to be aware of the risks and take precautions if work is being performed around such chemicals.

2.7: Botox—Does It Affect Pregnancy?

The recent discovery of Botox Cosmetic's magic has prompted many women to establish a routine of aesthetic Botox touch-ups, usually every 3–4 months. But what are the recommendations during pregnancy? Keep in mind that the onabotulinum toxin (also known as "Botox") is not used solely for wrinkles anymore. It is also being used to treat other medical conditions, such as migraine headaches and bladder dysfunction disorders. All of these uses have to be taken into consideration by the healthcare provider managing a pregnant woman. Therefore, the importance of reporting such uses of Botox (including the dosage amounts, frequency, and route of administration) to your healthcare provider is of utmost importance.

Botox and the Unborn Baby

While there is no concrete evidence suggesting it is totally safe, studies have not conclusively proven it is harmful either (Larson, 2020). Most healthcare providers advise putting Botox on hold until after pregnancy, just to play it safe.

If you are a Botox enthusiast facing pregnancy, it is a good idea to consult your healthcare provider. They can assist in weighing the risks, benefits, and uncertainties. Keep in mind that what suits one individual might not be suitable for someone else. It all comes down to making an informed choice that is compatible with your own pregnancy journey.

Therefore, when considering Botox and baby bumps, remember that it is a personal call. A healthcare provider can help in making a decision that keeps both mom-to-be and her little one safe and sound.

2.8: Prescription and Over-The-Counter (OTC) Medications During Pregnancy

When it comes to medications during pregnancy, there are two categories to consider: prescription and over-the-counter (OTC) medications.

1. **Prescription medications:** These are the ones that a doctor has prescribed for their patients. The managing OB doctor knows which prescription medications and dosages are safe for the mother and the baby; hence, it is important to take these medications as prescribed by the provider.
2. **OTC Medications:** These are medications that are bought without a prescription, such as pain relievers or cough syrup. It is important to emphasize here that not all OTC medications are safe to use during pregnancy, and this includes your herbal remedies and your self-prescribed, non-Rx nutritional supplements. It is a good idea to consult a doctor or a

pharmacist before taking anything, just to ensure it won't cause any problems for the coming baby.

Remember, self-care during pregnancy involves making smart choices about medications, too. A healthcare provider is a go-to resource for keeping both the mother and her baby safe and healthy.

Now that you have a comprehensive understanding of the potential vices, teratogens, and the impact of treatment medications on pregnancy, the next chapter will focus on the assessment of readiness for this transformative journey.

Chapter 3

Assessment of Readiness

3.1: Physical Fitness Before and During Pregnancy

Being active is more than just exercise—it is a way of life, a conscious lifestyle choice that involves caring for the body and overall well-being. Physical fitness can make a positive difference when a woman is planning for pregnancy or is already expecting.

Exercising Before Pregnancy

Staying active before pregnancy lays the groundwork for a smoother experience. Regular exercise can enhance overall health, help control weight, and even improve an expecting mom's mood—all valuable assets for what's to come. However, it is worth noting that there are times when achieving a specific weight range and activity level is not just beneficial, but also necessary and advised. This is particularly relevant when addressing pre-existing or potential medical concerns like obesity, diabetes, cardiac issues, and serious respiratory conditions. In these cases, attaining a recommended weight and activity level prior to conception is a wise move, bolstering the chances of a healthier pregnancy and better outcomes.

Exercising While Pregnant

Continuing to work out during pregnancy is recommended (NHS, 2023). Staying active during pregnancy can bring a variety of benefits, ranging from reducing discomfort to improving sleep. It's all about finding the right balance.

Tips for Exercising During Pregnancy

- **Attune to your body:** Give careful consideration to your physical sensations. If anything doesn't feel right, it's fine to slow down or modify exercises.
- **Stay hydrated:** Hydration is essential, so have that water bottle close.
- **Avoid overexertion:** Gentle exercises such as walking, swimming, and yoga can work wonders.
- **Choose supportive gear:** Wearing comfortable clothing and the right footwear can improve your comfort and safety.

Who Should Not Exercise While Pregnant

While exercise is great, certain situations do require caution:

- **High-risk pregnancy:** Consult a healthcare professional for issues such as preeclampsia or placenta previa.

- **Preterm labor history:** If a pregnant woman has previously experienced preterm labor, intense exercise may not be the best option.
- **Heart or lung issues:** Certain medical disorders may limit exercise options.

Examples of Some Safe Exercises During Pregnancy

- **Pelvic floor exercises:** Our body's secret superheroes! Exercises for your pelvis strengthen the muscles supporting the bladder, uterus, and bowels. You can prevent bladder leaks and help your body recover after giving birth by doing Kegel exercises, which include squeezing and holding these muscles (Mayo Clinic, 2022).
- **Pelvic tilt exercises:** You got a bit of backache? These exercises can come in handy. They alleviate lower back pain by gently tilting your pelvis forward and backward while on your hands and knees. It is like getting a mini-massage for your back!
- **Abdominal exercises:** The name of the game is to keep any abdominal exercises you do soft and gentle. While sit-ups might not be the best idea, you can perform gentle tummy tightening on your hands and knees. Strengthening tummy muscles can help to support a growing belly.

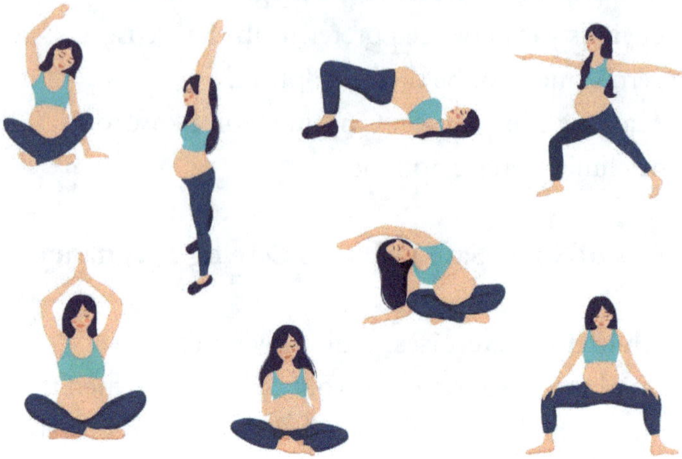

8 yoga exercises for pregnancy

Exercises That May Be Unsafe During Pregnancy

Certain exercises may require a rain check during pregnancy. For the following reasons:

- **Heavy lifting:** Your muscles and ligaments are putting in a lot of effort to support your baby. Lifting heavy weights can be taxing on them and might not be the best choice.
- **Contact sports:** As much as you enjoy a good game, popular contact sports such as soccer, basketball, volleyball, or boxing can put you in danger of falling or getting hit. Your body is in superhero mode, but it's best to avoid these intense games for now.
- **High-impact activities:** Think twice about activities that require a lot of jumping or sudden

changes in direction. Your balance is changing, and these moves can be dangerous.
- **Scuba diving:** While underwater excursions sound exciting, the pressure and lack of oxygen may be harmful to your baby.
- **Avoid lying flat on your back after 16 weeks of gestation:** From 16 weeks of gestation onward, it is recommended that pregnant women avoid lying flat on their back for prolonged periods. This is because the pressure of the baby's weight on the major blood vessels supplying the heart and the brain may create flow obstruction, resulting in dizziness and fainting (NHS, 2023d).

The following categories of pregnant women should not be routinely exercising without a doctor's preapproval or guidance: Women with a history of past miscarriage(s), weak cervix, low-lying placenta, and premature labor or birth. Remember, your health and the safety of your baby come first. If you have any doubts regarding an exercise, consult your healthcare provider. The goal is to find the right balance between staying active and staying safe.

3.2: Emotional Readiness for Pregnancy

Pregnancy affects not only physical health aspects but also emotional well-being. Here's a glimpse into how to emotionally prepare for the wonderful journey ahead:

- **Understanding personal feelings:** It's normal to feel a mix of excitement, anxiety, and even dread.

Recognize that all of these feelings are a part of the process.

- **Acquire knowledge:** Knowledge is empowering. Gather as much knowledge as you can about pregnancy, childbirth, and the journey into parenthood. This can minimize uncertainties and enhance confidence.
- **Self-care:** Take time for yourself. Pamper yourself to alleviate stress by reading, listening to music, or taking a warm bath.
- **Preparing for change:** Pregnancy transforms not just the female body, but also her life. These adjustments should be accepted with an open heart and a positive attitude.
- **Letting go of perfection:** Nobody is a perfect parent. Accept that mistakes can happen and concentrate on doing better.
- **Mindfulness and relaxation:** Practice techniques like meditation and deep breathing to gain stability and relaxation. These practices have become popular in recent times, and there is an abundance of ebooks and audible books available for purchase and sometimes for free on online marketplace platforms such as Amazon and Google Books.

Remember that it is okay to have emotions. Your emotions as a mom-to-be are considered valid and genuine, regardless of whether they are positive or negative. Accept them and allow them to guide you through this amazing journey of emotional readiness for pregnancy.

3.3: Evaluating Your Support Systems

Having a strong support system throughout pregnancy can make all the difference. Here are some tips for assessing and strengthening your support network:

- **Family and friends:** Observe the people around you. Who can you rely on for emotional support, practical help, and encouragement? Consider your friends and family members who are always there for you, and don't hesitate to reach out to them.
- **Partner:** Your partner's role in this journey cannot be overlooked. Open communication is necessary. Discuss your needs, fears, and expectations. This is a time for teamwork and understanding.
- **Healthcare provider:** Your doctor or midwife is an important part of your support network. Are you at ease asking questions and discussing concerns? A caring healthcare provider can help you overcome your worries.
- **Online and offline groups:** Joining pregnancy groups, either in person or online, can link you with other expectant mothers who understand what you're going through. Sharing experiences and advice can be comforting.
- **Workplace and maternity leave:** Review your workplace's policies on maternity leave and flexibility. Knowing your options can help you prepare for an easier transition.
- **Parenting classes:** Enrolling in prenatal classes can

provide a wealth of information and an opportunity to connect with other parents-to-be.

- **Financial support:** Assess your financial status and plan for any adjustments required during pregnancy and after childbirth.
- **Emergency contacts:** Keep a record of essential emergency contacts for quick access.
- **Mental health support:** If you have a history of mental health issues, make sure you have access to proper help during your pregnancy.

Go ahead and ask for help when necessary. Building and cultivating a strong support network can pave the way for a more positive and fulfilling pregnancy experience.

Now that you are armed with insights regarding your own readiness, get ready to delve into the fascinating stages that lie ahead. The next chapter explores the transformative path that leads from conception to the milestones of each trimester.

Part Two

Conception, Early Pregnancy, and the Trimesters

Whether your pregnancy was meticulously planned, medically coaxed, or happened by surprise, one thing is certain—your life will never be the same.

— Catherine Jones

Chapter 4

In the Beginning

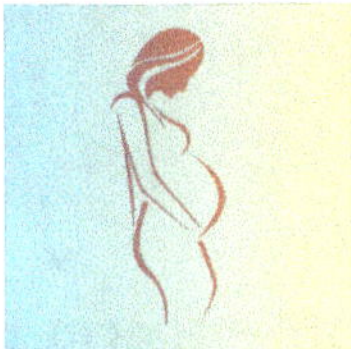

From the moment of conception to the delicate early days of pregnancy and the changing trimesters that follow, each moment highlights the amazing process of human creation. Get ready to delve into the fascinating story of how new life begins, grows, and the journey that shapes the start of motherhood.

4.1: From Conception/Fertilization to Implantation

Human life begins with the fusion of a single egg cell and a sperm cell. Fertilization, also known as conception, normally occurs within the fallopian tubes. It is here that the genetic material from both parents unites to form the new individual's unique and full set of DNA.

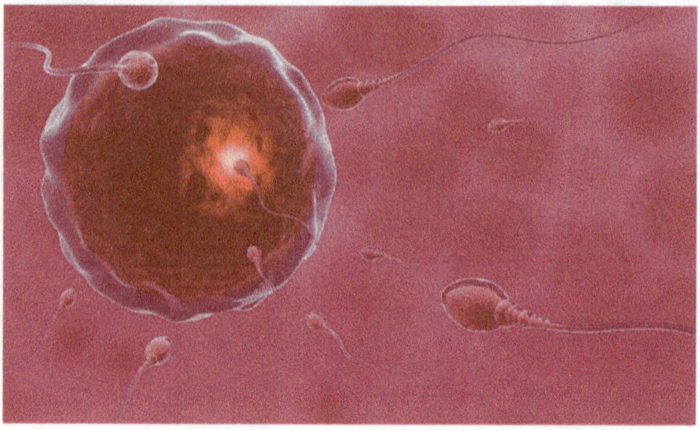

Fertilization – sperm-egg fusion

Counting weeks: Interestingly, the way pregnancy weeks are counted may come as a surprise. While it is commonly believed that pregnancy begins at conception, medically, the first day of pregnancy is considered to be the first day of your last menstrual period (LMP). This difference occurs because it is often challenging to pinpoint the exact day of conception. Therefore, when a woman is around two to three weeks past conception, doctors consider her to be four to five weeks pregnant, according to the LMP.

Implantation and the embryo: After conception, the fertilized egg divides rapidly as it travels down the fallopian tube toward the uterus. The embryo enters the uterus 6–10 days after fertilization, and the implantation process begins. This involves the embryo attaching itself to the blood-rich uterine lining, where it will receive nourishment and develop over the next few weeks.

Early pregnancy signs: During these crucial first weeks, the mother's body might begin displaying some subtle signs of pregnancy. Hormonal changes can cause tender breasts, slight fatigue, and even mild mood swings. However, these signs are easily overlooked or attributed to other causes, so many women remain unaware of their pregnancy at this point.

A hidden miracle: The first couple of weeks, marked by fertilization and implantation, are full of extraordinary biological events that set the stage for the growth and development of the tiny embryo. It's only after these initial weeks have passed that pregnancy tests can identify the presence of the pregnancy hormone hCG (human chorionic gonadotropin) in the mother's urine, increasing the likelihood that she is pregnant.

4.2: When Implantation Goes Wrong: Ectopic Pregnancy and Early Miscarriage

Implantation plays a key role in the early stages of pregnancy. However, in some cases, implantation can go wrong, leading to ectopic pregnancy and early miscarriage. These complications can be distressing and need prompt medical attention.

Ectopic Pregnancy

An ectopic pregnancy occurs when the fertilized egg implants outside the uterus, usually in the fallopian tubes. This condition is not viable and can pose serious health risks for the pregnant woman.

Symptoms

- abdominal pain, usually on one side
- vaginal bleeding
- shoulder pain (caused by internal bleeding)
- feeling faint or dizzy

- pain with bowel movements or urination

Treatment

- ultrasound and blood testing for early detection
- medication (methotrexate) inhibits cell growth and dissolves the pregnancy (Abdulkareem & Eidan, 2017)
- surgical removal of the ectopic pregnancy or damaged fallopian tube
- regular monitoring and follow-up care

Early Miscarriage (Spontaneous Abortion)

An early miscarriage occurs when a pregnancy is lost within the first 20 weeks. It can result from various factors, including chromosomal abnormalities and health problems.

Symptoms

- vaginal bleeding, mostly with clots
- abdominal cramps
- tissue passing through the vagina
- diminishing pregnancy symptoms (breast tenderness, nausea)
- back pain

Treatment

- there will be no treatment if the miscarriage is unavoidable and complete

- medication to end a miscarriage (medical management)
- dilation and curettage (D&C) techniques to remove residual tissue (surgical management) (Mayo Clinic, 2021)
- emotional support and post-treatment monitoring

Prevention and Seeking Help

- early prenatal care to monitor pregnancy health
- awareness of risk factors, such as previous ectopic pregnancies or miscarriages
- seeking medical attention for any odd symptoms
- open discussions with healthcare providers about prior gynecological history and problems

Shared Considerations

- Both ectopic pregnancies and early miscarriages involve failed implantation of the embryo.
- Early detection through regular prenatal care and communication with healthcare providers is essential.
- Emotional support and counseling are necessary for women experiencing these situations.

Understanding, diagnosis, and treatment options for ectopic pregnancies and early miscarriages continue to improve due to research and medical advancements (Sivalingam et al., 2011).

Remember that medical information is subject to change and should be reviewed by a competent healthcare professional for the most accurate and up-to-date advice.

4.3: How to Recognize the Early Signs of Pregnancy; Pregnancy Testing Home Kits; Pregnancy Testing By Blood

Recognizing the early signs of pregnancy are essential for proper management and planning. Home pregnancy tests and blood tests are reliable methods to confirm pregnancy. Here's a quick guide:

Early Signs of Pregnancy

- **Missed period:** A missed period is one of the most common signs of pregnancy.
- **Breast changes:** Increased tenderness and/or pain, swelling, or darkening of the areolas.
- **Fatigue:** Excessive tiredness caused by hormonal changes.
- **Nausea and vomiting:** Also known as morning sickness (hyperemesis gravidarum), can occur at any time of day.
- **Frequent urge to urinate:** Hormonal changes increase blood flow to the pelvic area.
- **Food aversions and cravings:** These are defined as sudden dislikes or strong urges for eating certain foods.
- **Mood swings:** Hormonal fluctuations can cause emotional changes.

Home Pregnancy Tests

- **How they work:** They work by detecting the hCG hormone in urine.
- **When to take:** For accurate results, wait until after a missed period.
- **Accuracy:** When used properly, accuracy is high; some tests can detect pregnancy even before a missed period.
- **Instructions:** Follow the package directions carefully for the best results. Be sure to always check the expiration date for every home pregnancy kit prior to purchase and prior to use.
- **Result interpretation:** Positive (two lines or a digital "pregnant") or negative (one line or "not pregnant").

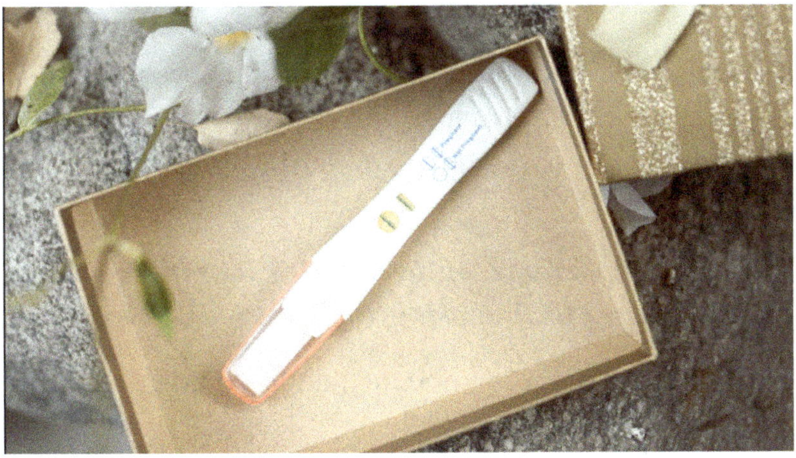

Positive pregnancy test – two lines

Blood Pregnancy Tests

- **Types:** Qualitative blood test (confirms pregnancy) and quantitative blood test (measures hCG levels).
- **Accuracy:** Excellent; can detect very low levels of hCG.
- **Timing:** This can be performed as early as 7–12 days following fertilization, which is sooner than home tests.
- **Procedure:** A blood sample is obtained and delivered to a lab at a healthcare facility for testing.
- **Result interpretation:** A positive result confirms pregnancy and hCG levels can indicate the stage of pregnancy.
- **Consult a healthcare professional:** Discuss your results with a doctor to properly understand your pregnancy's progress.

Remember that everyone's experience is unique, and not all women experience the same symptoms. If you suspect you are pregnant, seek proper testing and advice from a healthcare expert.

4.4: The Importance of Prenatal Vitamins in Early Pregnancy and the Importance of the Prenatal Visit

Prenatal care plays an important role in ensuring a healthy pregnancy and successful childbirth. Prenatal vitamins and regular prenatal visits are essential components of this care, especially during the early stages of pregnancy. These practices are intended to promote the well-being of both the expectant mother and the developing fetus.

Importance of Prenatal Vitamins in Early Pregnancy

- **Nutritional support:** Prenatal vitamins are specially formulated to supply key nutrients necessary for fetal development and maternal health.
- **Folic acid:** Folic acid in prenatal supplements helps prevent neural tube defects and supports early embryonic growth.
- **Iron and calcium:** Adequate iron promotes blood production, while calcium promotes the development of the baby's bones and teeth.
- **Vitamin D:** Vitamin D is essential for bone health and immune system function and is frequently included in prenatal supplements.
- **Iodine:** Iodine is essential for thyroid function and brain development, and it is especially vital for the baby's cognitive development.

Importance of Prenatal Visits

- **Monitoring health:** Prenatal checkups allow healthcare experts to monitor the mother's health and treat any potential concerns.
- **Fetal development:** Regular check-ups allow for the monitoring of fetal growth, heart rate, and overall well-being. Your healthcare provider will measure fundal height during your visits. Fundal height measurement is the distance from the pubic bone up to the top of your uterus during pregnancy (Neilson, 1998). This important measurement serves two main purposes: Initially, it assists the healthcare provider in

assessing the fetus's proper development, and subsequently, it contributes to determining the gestational age, indicating the progress of the pregnancy.

- **Early detection:** Prenatal checkups aid in the early detection and management of medical conditions such as gestational diabetes and preeclampsia.
- **Education and guidance:** Healthcare experts provide vital information on nutrition, exercise, and labor and birthing preparation.
- **Emotional support:** Prenatal visits provide an opportunity for expectant women to discuss their physical and emotional experiences.

4.5: The Trimesters

The word "trimester" is the medical term for describing how pregnancy is organized. Pregnancy is divided into three trimesters, each of which lasts for around three months. Here's a brief overview of each trimester.

First Trimester (Month 1–3)

This is the first stage of pregnancy when the body undergoes considerable changes as it adjusts to the growing fetus.

- **Weeks 1–4:** Although conception usually begins around week 2, the first week is recorded from the last menstrual cycle. The fertilized egg implants in the uterus and starts dividing rapidly.
- **Weeks 5–8:** The embryo's primary organs and systems, including the heart, brain, spinal cord, and

limbs, begin to form. Common symptoms include morning nausea, breast discomfort, and exhaustion.
- **Weeks 9–12,** The embryo is now referred to as a fetus. The fetus's facial features become more distinct and it begins to move. Miscarriage risk diminishes, and the placenta takes over hormone production.

Second Trimester (Month 4–6)

This trimester is often considered the most comfortable period of pregnancy, as many early pregnancy symptoms tend to subside.

- **Weeks 13–16:** The fetus undergoes rapid growth. Gender can usually be determined, and the baby's skin is transparent. The mother might feel the first flutters of fetal movement.
- **Weeks 17–20:** The mother can feel clearer movements, and the fetus's senses begin to develop. Vernix, a natural protective coating, develops on the surface of the skin.
- **Weeks 21–24:** The fetus's lungs continue to grow, making survival outside of the womb possible. The fetus develops eyebrows and eyelashes and can respond to external sounds (LDH, n.d.).

Third Trimester (Month 7–9)

This is the final stage of pregnancy, characterized by the fetus's continued growth and the final preparations for birth.

- **Weeks 25–28:** The fetus's brain is rapidly developing, and the eyes can open and close. Lung development continues, and the fetus gains more body fat.
- **Weeks 29–32:** The fetus's bones are fully formed but still soft. The baby's movements might feel stronger and more defined. The mother's uterus might cause more discomfort.
- **Weeks 33–36:** In preparation for birth, the fetus settles into a head-down position. As the mother's body prepares for birth, she may experience more frequent Braxton-Hicks contractions. These contractions are commonly known as "practice contractions" because they are sporadic and irregular tightening of the uterine muscles. The uterus uses these contractions to prepare and tone the muscles for labor and delivery. Braxton-Hicks contractions, unlike genuine labor contractions, are usually painless and do not indicate the start of active labor.
- **Weeks 37–40 (full-term):** The baby is considered full-term at 37 weeks. The fetus's organs are fully developed, and it is ready for life outside the womb. Labor normally begins between weeks 38–42.

Pregnancy timeframes can vary, making regular prenatal care necessary for both mother and baby's health. The next chapter explores the early stages of pregnancy, where the incredible transformation journey begins. It digs into the intricate details of this remarkable initial phase.

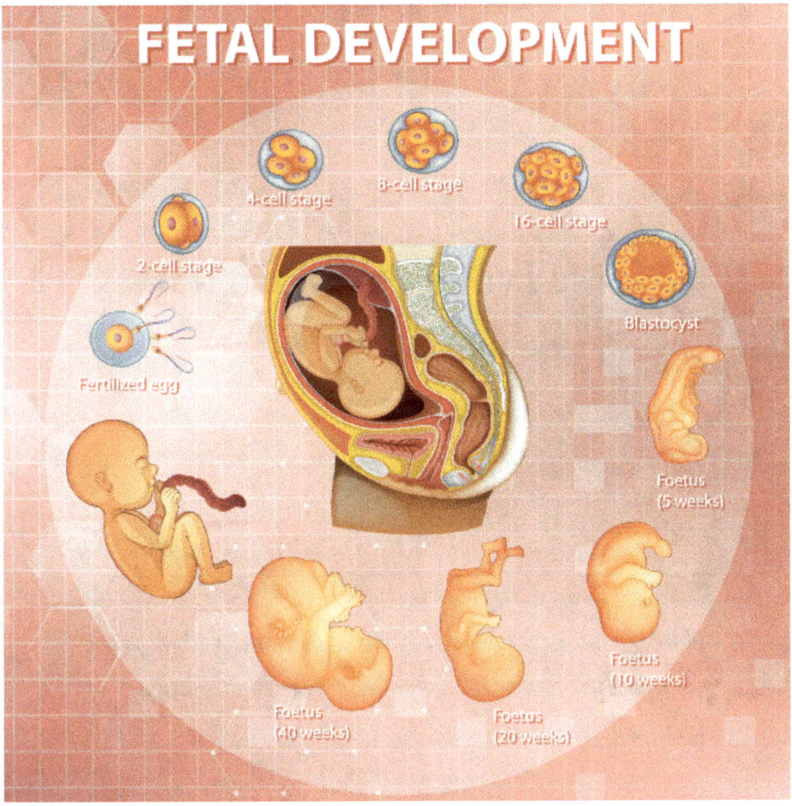
FETAL DEVELOPMENT
Fertilized egg
2-cell stage
4-cell stage
8-cell stage
16-cell stage
Blastocyst
Foetus
(5 weeks)
Foetus
(10 weeks)
Foetus
(20 weeks)
Foetus
(40 weeks)

First Trimester Overview

Motherhood is the biggest gamble in the world. It is the glorious life force. It's huge and scary—it's an act of infinite optimism.

— Gilda Radner

The first trimester of pregnancy marks the beginning of a fascinating journey packed with profound changes and expectations. It is a key stage for both mother and baby, during which certain habits need to be adjusted, potential risks managed, and common symptoms addressed. This section delves into key aspects of the first trimester, ranging from lifestyle adjustments to understanding symptoms and managing unexpected concerns.

Time to change some habits. Expectant women often find themselves making important lifestyle changes during the first trimester of pregnancy, especially in cases of unplanned pregnancies. Details of this have already been discussed in Chapter 2.

First trimester symptoms and how to manage them. The first trimester usually arrives with a host of symptoms that may be challenging for expectant mothers. Nausea and vomiting, fatigue, appetite changes, drowsiness, and breast tenderness are common occurrences. To alleviate these discomforts, it's advisable to eat smaller, more frequent meals, remain hydrated, relax as required, and wear a supportive bra. Consulting with a healthcare provider can also offer advice on how to properly manage these symptoms.

Bleeding/spotting in the first trimester. Experiencing bleeding or spotting during the first trimester can be a cause for concern for pregnant women. Although it is not always a sign of alarm, it is essential to understand the possible implications (American College of Obstetricians and Gynecologists, 2021). The bleeding can vary from light spotting, which is only a few drops of blood, to heavy bleeding that resembles a period. If you experience any bleeding or spotting, it is essential to keep the following factors in mind:

- **Implantation bleeding:** Light bleeding or spotting occurring around the time of your expected period could be due to the embryo attaching itself to the uterine lining. This is generally harmless and may last for a day or two.

- **Miscarriage:** Unfortunately, bleeding can sometimes signal a miscarriage, especially if it is accompanied by severe abdominal pain and cramping. Seek emergency medical help if you think you are having a miscarriage.
- **Ectopic pregnancy:** Sometimes, bleeding may be a sign of an ectopic pregnancy, as already explained in Chapter 4. Ectopic pregnancies are dangerous and demand urgent medical attention.
- **Cervical changes:** Sometimes, minor bleeding can occur due to changes in the cervix during pregnancy. This is usually harmless.
- **Other causes:** Bleeding can result from other factors like cervical irritation, infections, or cervical polyps (tiny, harmless growths or lumps that can appear on the cervix).

Keep in mind that it is crucial not to ignore any bleeding or spotting throughout the first trimester. Get in touch with your healthcare provider, describe your symptoms in detail, and follow their advice. To safeguard your health and the well-being of your unborn baby, they may recommend tests, ultrasounds, or other procedures. Remember that early detection and prompt medical intervention can make a significant difference in the outcome.

Chapter 5

Pregnancy Month 1 (Weeks 3–6)

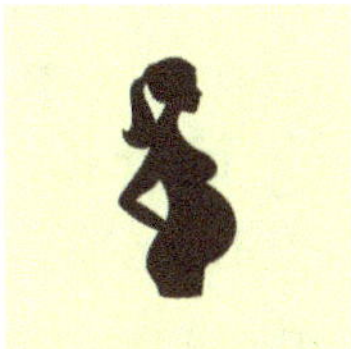

The first month of pregnancy, spanning from weeks 3 to 6, marks the earliest stage of pregnancy and is often characterized by a combination of excitement and trepidation. The developing fetus is incredibly small, measuring just a few millimeters in length. Many of the crucial developmental milestones cannot yet be observed in medical imaging, and the exact timing of these processes can vary from one pregnancy to another.

Furthermore, expectant mothers may encounter a variety of early signs and symptoms, some of which can be rather difficult. Three common symptoms in this initial phase of pregnancy include morning sickness, fatigue, and breast tenderness. Keep reading to discover the reasons behind these sensations, dispel myths surrounding them, and learn practical strategies for managing them.

5.1: Early Signs and Symptoms

Morning Sickness: "Why Am I so Queasy?"

Morning sickness, contrary to its deceptive title, has the potential to manifest at various times throughout the day. Hormonal changes, specifically higher levels of hCG, are to blame for this symptom. Contrary to popular belief, morning sickness does not necessarily indicate a healthy pregnancy, nor does its absence signal a problem (Danielsson, 2021). Not all women experience morning sickness, and the severity varies greatly.

To alleviate morning sickness, consider eating smaller, more frequent meals to avoid an empty stomach, avoiding trigger foods or smells, and staying hydrated. Ginger, vitamin B6 supplements, and acupressure wristbands are also possible treatments that may help. Consult with a healthcare provider if morning sickness becomes severe, as this can lead to dehydration or weight loss.

Fatigue: "I Just Want to Sleep."

The extreme exhaustion felt during the first trimester is mostly due to an increase in progesterone, a hormone that induces relaxation and can leave you feeling completely drained. This exhaustion might be exacerbated by the mental and physical changes that occur in your body as it prepares to nurture a growing fetus.

Prioritizing rest and sleep are crucial for combating weariness. This may imply changing your daily schedule to allow for more naps or an earlier bedtime. Prenatal yoga, for example, can help raise energy levels. Additionally, eating a well-balanced, nutrient-dense diet can help to alleviate fatigue.

Breast Tenderness: "My Nipples Hurt."

Breast tenderness and sensitivity are prevalent in early pregnancy as a result of hormonal changes, particularly an increase in estrogen and progesterone. Soreness and pain might result from increased blood flow and preparation of the mammary glands for breastfeeding.

To alleviate breast tenderness, choose a supportive, comfortable bra, preferably one without an underwire. Applying warm compresses or taking a warm bath can provide relief. Avoiding harsh soaps and detergents that may irritate the skin in this sensitive area is also advisable.

5.2: Confirmation of Pregnancy

Pregnancy confirmation usually involves several methods and steps. Here is an overview of how pregnancy is typically confirmed.

- **Home Pregnancy Test (HPT):** The most commonly used method for confirming pregnancy is to use a home pregnancy test. These tests detect the presence of the pregnancy hormone, hCG, in the urine. HPTs are readily available in most drugstores and can be used as soon as a few days after a missed period. They are generally believed to be accurate when used correctly.
- **Blood test:** If you have a positive result on a home pregnancy test, it's usually a good idea to follow up

with a blood test administered by a healthcare provider. A blood test measures the level of hCG in your blood, providing a more precise indication of pregnancy, and can detect pregnancy earlier than a urine test. Blood tests can also be used to estimate the duration of a pregnancy.

- **Clinical assessment:** After receiving a positive result on a home pregnancy test or blood test, it is necessary to schedule an appointment with a healthcare provider, such as an obstetrician or gynecologist. During this appointment, your healthcare provider will review your medical history, perform a physical examination, and request additional tests or ultrasounds to confirm the pregnancy and determine the health of the fetus.
- **Ultrasound:** An ultrasound is a useful tool for confirming and monitoring pregnancy. While it is not usually used as the main method of confirmation, it can reveal important information such as the pregnancy's location, viability, and gestational age. An early ultrasound, typically performed between six and eight weeks of pregnancy, can confirm the presence of a developing embryo or fetus and may be used if the pregnancy is causing any concerns.
- **Additional testing:** In some cases, further testing may be necessary to evaluate the progress of the pregnancy or assess any potential complications. This may include additional blood tests, genetic screening, or specialized diagnostic procedures based on the individual's health and medical history.

It's important to remember that a single negative result on a home pregnancy test does not definitively rule out pregnancy, especially if it is done too early in the pregnancy or if the test is not handled correctly. If there are any doubts or worries about a pregnancy, it is advisable to consult with a healthcare provider for a thorough evaluation and appropriate guidance.

5.3: Little Things That Matter Now

Why Is My Cat a Problem Now?

The beloved feline companion in your life can bring comfort and joy, but during pregnancy, it's essential to be aware of potential risks associated with your cat.

Toxoplasmosis risk: Pregnant women need to be cautious about handling cat litter as it can contain the toxoplasma parasite, which can be harmful to the developing fetus.

Infection prevention: To prevent toxoplasmosis, pregnant individuals should wear gloves when changing cat litter, wash their hands thoroughly afterward, and consider having someone else handle litter duty if possible.

Indoor cats: Keeping cats indoors can reduce the risk of exposure to toxoplasma since indoor cats are less likely to be infected than outdoor cats.

The Dangers of Deli Meats

Listeria risk: Deli meats, like cold cuts and hot dogs, can potentially carry *listeria* bacteria, which can cause serious complications during pregnancy, including miscarriage, preterm birth, or stillbirth.

Safe handling: Pregnant women should heat deli meats until steaming hot to destroy any harmful bacteria, rather than eating them cold.

Alternative proteins: To prevent the risks associated with deli meats, consider using alternative protein sources such as cooked poultry or vegetarian options.

The Lurking Perils in Gardening

Gardening may be a rewarding and calming pastime for pregnant women, but they should be aware of potential hazards and take care to safeguard their safety and the health of their unborn child. Here are some of the lurking perils in gardening for pregnant women:

Soil-borne pathogens: Soil can host a variety of dangerous microorganisms, including bacteria like E. coli and *salmonella*, which can cause gastrointestinal infections if ingested.

Preventive measures:

- Wear gardening gloves to avoid having direct contact with soil.
- Thoroughly wash hands with soap and water after gardening to remove any soil or contaminants.
- Avoid touching your face, particularly your mouth, nose, and eyes, while gardening.

Chemical exposure: The use of pesticides, herbicides, and fertilizers in gardening can expose people to potentially toxic chemicals, some of which are detrimental to pregnant women and their babies.

Preventive measures:

- Choose natural or organic pesticides and herbicides instead of chemical alternatives.
- If it is necessary to use chemical products, wear protective clothing, including gloves and a mask, and ensure proper ventilation.
- After handling chemicals, wash properly and wait for the recommended period before returning to the garden.

Heavy lifting and physical strain: Overexertion, heavy lifting, or unexpected intense exercise can be dangerous, particularly in late pregnancy.

Preventive measures:

- Lifting large objects or indulging in strenuous tasks should be avoided.
- To reduce the need for bending and lifting, use ergonomic tools and raised garden beds.
- Take frequent rests and pay attention to your body's signals of exhaustion or discomfort.

Dehydration and overheating: Gardening in the sun in hot weather can cause dehydration and overheating (hyperthermia), both of which are dangerous for pregnant women.

Preventive measures:

- Drink plenty of water throughout your gardening session to stay hydrated.

- Garden during cooler times of the day to stay safe from excessive heat exposure.
- To shield yourself from the sun, dress in light, breezy clothing and a wide-brimmed hat.

5.4: Your Baby's Developmental Milestones in the First 4 Weeks

In the first four weeks of pregnancy, which is often referred to as the embryonic period, a series of remarkable developmental milestones occur within the womb (uterus). It's worth mentioning that during this early stage, many of these milestones happen on a microscopic level, but they lay the foundation for the development of a healthy baby. Here are the key developmental milestones during this period:

Week 1: Fertilization and Implantation

- **Fertilization:** The sperm and egg combine in the fallopian tube, resulting in the formation of a single-celled zygote.
- **Journey to the uterus:** The zygote begins its journey from the fallopian tube to the uterus.
- **Implantation:** By the end of the first week, the zygote reaches the uterus and implants into the uterine lining. Now, it is referred to as a blastocyst (Artal-Mittelmark, 2022).

Week 2: Formation of the Embryo

- **Formation of germ layers:** The blastocyst divides into three germ layers (ectoderm, mesoderm, and endoderm), from which various organs and tissues will emerge.

- **Formation of the amniotic sac:** The amniotic sac, which will protect and cushion the developing embryo, starts to form.

Week 3: Beginning of Organ Development

- **Formation of neural tube:** The neural tube, which will eventually become the brain and spinal cord, starts developing.
- **Primitive heart:** The heart begins to develop and beat, but it is still just a basic tube.

Week 4: Rapid Growth and Heartbeat

- **Rapid growth:** The embryo undergoes significant growth and acquires a more recognizable shape.
- **Formation of major organs:** Organs and structures, including the heart, blood vessels, liver, and primitive circulatory system, continue developing.
- **Heartbeat:** By the end of week 4, the heart's electrical activity produces the first detectable heartbeat, though it is still a tiny, flickering pulse.

By the end of the fourth week, your baby's size will be comparable to that of a tiny grain of rice! The significance of B vitamins cannot be overstated in supporting both your and your baby's growth and maintaining your health throughout pregnancy. Specifically, Vitamin B6 and Folic Acid (Vitamin B9) hold great importance in the early stages of development, so it's essential to ensure you are receiving appropriate quantities of these nutrients (American Pregnancy Association, n.d.-b).

5.5: The First Prenatal Visit and What to Expect

The first prenatal visit is an important stage in the journey of pregnancy. During this appointment, you will meet with a healthcare provider, usually an obstetrician or midwife, to initiate prenatal care and ensure the health and well-being of both you and your baby. Here's what you can generally expect during your first prenatal visit:

- **Medical history review:** Your healthcare provider will begin by taking a detailed medical history. This includes your personal and family medical history, as well as any past pregnancies and their results.
- **Physical examination:** This may include checking your weight, blood pressure, and heart rate. Your provider may also examine your breasts, abdomen, and pelvis.
- **Pelvic exam and Pap smear:** Depending on your specific situation and previous medical history, your healthcare provider may perform a pelvic exam and a Pap smear (cervical cell sample for testing) to check for any cervical abnormalities.
- **Pelvic ultrasound:** In some cases, particularly if you are unsure about the gestational age of your pregnancy, a pelvic ultrasound may be performed to assess how far along you are and confirm the pregnancy.

- **Blood and urine tests:** Blood tests will be conducted to determine your blood type and Rh factor and check for conditions such as anemia, infections, and sexually transmitted infections (STIs). Urine tests may also be performed to check for signs of kidney or urinary tract issues.
- **Discussion of symptoms and concerns:** This is an opportunity for you to discuss any symptoms, concerns, or questions you may have regarding your pregnancy, including morning sickness, fatigue, or weird feelings.
- **Prenatal vitamins and medications:** Your healthcare provider may recommend or prescribe prenatal vitamins containing folic acid, which is necessary for fetal development. They will also review any current medications you are taking and advise you on their safety during pregnancy.
- **Discussion of lifestyle and habits:** You will be asked about your lifestyle and habits, such as your diet, exercise routine, smoking, alcohol consumption, and exposure to environmental hazards. Your healthcare provider will offer guidance on making healthy decisions during pregnancy.
- **Establishing a prenatal care schedule:** Your provider will outline the schedule for your prenatal care appointments. You will usually have regular check-ups throughout your pregnancy, with visits becoming more frequent as your due date approaches.
- **Pregnancy education:** Your first prenatal visit also provides the opportunity to receive educational

resources and information about prenatal classes, nutrition, and what to expect during each trimester of your pregnancy.

- **Discussion of the birth plan and delivery preferences:** Depending on your healthcare provider's practice, you may be able to discuss your labor and delivery preferences, such as choosing between a hospital birth and a birthing center.
- **Next steps:** Your healthcare provider will guide you on what to expect in the coming weeks and how to schedule future appointments and tests.

Keep in mind that every prenatal care visit may vary depending on your individual requirements and medical history.

5.6: Pregnancy Blood Work for Prenatal Screening

Pregnancy blood work for prenatal screening is an essential part of prenatal care, aimed at assessing the mother's health and identifying any potential risks or conditions that might affect the pregnancy. Here's a breakdown of some common blood tests performed during pregnancy:

- **Complete blood count (CBC):** Monitors the levels of various blood components.
- **Relevance in pregnancy:** Helps detect anemia (low red blood cell count) and possible infections or inflammation (high white blood cell count).
- **Complete metabolic panel (CMP):** Measures glucose levels, electrolytes, and liver and kidney function.

- **Relevance in pregnancy:** Checks blood sugar levels (essential for gestational diabetes monitoring) and ensures that the liver and kidneys are functioning properly.
- **Rhesus factor (Rh Factor):** Determines whether or not the Rh factor is present in a person's blood.
- **Relevance in pregnancy:** Rh factor compatibility between the mother and baby is crucial. If the mother is Rh-negative and the baby is Rh-positive, there is a risk of Rh incompatibility, which can cause hemolytic disease in the newborn (HDN). Rhogam injections may be recommended to prevent sensitization.
- **Hepatitis B screening:** Identifies the presence of the hepatitis B virus in the mother's blood.
- **Relevance in pregnancy:** Identifying hepatitis B infection is important because it can be passed from the mother to her baby during childbirth. If the mother is infected, steps can be taken to lower the risk of transmission to the newborn, such as administering hepatitis B immune globulin and the hepatitis B vaccine.
- **Sickle cell trait and disease screening:** Detects the presence of sickle cell trait or sickle cell illness in the mother's blood.
- **Relevance in pregnancy:** If a mother has sickle cell trait or illness, it is essential to monitor the pregnancy closely, as it can lead to complications. Additionally, knowing the status of the parents helps determine the risk of passing the trait or illness to the baby.

5.7. Physical Changes

There are several physical changes and developments taking place in a woman's body as the pregnancy begins to take shape. These changes are generally minor at this early stage but are essential for the healthy progression of pregnancy. Some of the key physical changes include

- **Missed period:** This is one of the earliest signs of pregnancy. This occurs because the body has begun producing human chorionic gonadotropin (hCG), a hormone that stops the shedding of the uterine lining, resulting in a missed period.
- **Increased urination:** Hormonal changes can also result in increased urination. The uterus can put pressure on the bladder, leading to frequent trips to the bathroom.
- **Changes in cervical mucus:** Hormonal fluctuations can cause changes in cervical mucus. It may become thicker and stickier, forming a mucus plug that protects the uterus from infection.
- **Implantation bleeding:** Some women may experience minor spotting or bleeding around the time of embryo implantation. This is usually shorter and lighter than a normal menstrual cycle.
- **Basal body temperature:** Body temperature may remain high due to enhanced progesterone production.
- **Uterine changes:** The uterus may undergo subtle changes as it prepares for pregnancy. It may become slightly enlarged and softer.

It is worth mentioning that not all women will experience these physical changes to the same extent, and some may not experience them at all. Also, many of these changes are triggered by hormonal fluctuations and the body's preparations for pregnancy. If you suspect you are pregnant or have concerns about physical changes during early pregnancy, you should seek advice and confirmation from a healthcare provider.

5.8: Emotional Changes

Emotional changes can be considerable as women navigate the early stages of pregnancy. While each person has their own experience, here are some common emotional changes and challenges that may arise at this time:

- **Excitement:** Many women feel a sense of excitement and joy when they first discover they're pregnant. The prospect of being a parent and bringing new life into the world can be thrilling.
- **Anxiety:** Alongside excitement, anxiety is also common. The first trimester is a period of uncertainty. Many expectant mothers worry about their baby's health, potential difficulties, and their ability to handle the responsibilities of motherhood.
- **Nervousness:** Fear of the unknown can contribute to uneasy feelings. It's natural to have questions and concerns about the changes that are coming and how they will affect one's life.
- **Mood swings:** Hormonal fluctuations play an important role in emotional changes during early pregnancy. These hormonal shifts can cause mood

swings, making a pregnant woman feel happy one moment and tearful or irritable the next.

- **Apprehension:** Women may be concerned about sharing the news of their pregnancy with loved ones or their employers. The timing and circumstances of the pregnancy can influence how one approaches these conversations.
- **Bonding:** Some women may begin to feel a bond with the developing fetus at this time, while others might take longer. The emotional connection with the baby may get stronger as the pregnancy progresses.
- **Changes in body image:** Early physical changes, like breast tenderness and bloating, can affect how a woman sees her body. This could lead to conflicting feelings about one's body image.
- **Fatigue:** The increased fatigue common during the first trimester can have an effect on emotional well-being. Feeling tired can make it difficult to cope with stress or effectively control emotions.
- **Acceptance:** As the reality of pregnancy sinks in, many women gradually learn to accept the changes and uncertainties that come with it, resulting in a more stable emotional state.

During the first trimester of pregnancy, it is normal to experience emotional changes and expectant mothers are encouraged to prioritize self-care and seek help from healthcare providers and loved ones. As the initial excitement and challenges of the first-month fade, the second month marks a turning point in the pregnancy journey, with significant developments and milestones for both the mother and the growing baby.

Chapter 6

Pregnancy Month 2 (Weeks 7–10)

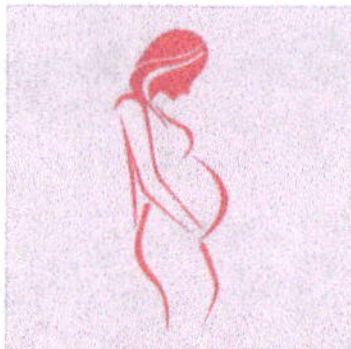

The second month of pregnancy is a period of profound changes and exciting milestones. As your journey continues, you'll witness significant developments in your baby's growth and experience further physical and emotional transformations. This chapter navigates the key aspects of the second month, from the blossoming of your baby's features to the evolving experiences of expectant mothers.

6.1: Your Baby's Developmental Milestones in the Second Month

This is a crucial period for fetal development, as many vital structures and systems begin to form. It's essential for the mother to continue to eat well to support her health and provide essential nutrients for the growing baby.

The following are some key developmental milestones.

Week 7

- **Heartbeat:** By the end of the seventh week, the baby's heart is normally functioning and may be detectable through ultrasound.
- **Brain development:** The brain continues to grow and develop with the formation of the cerebral hemispheres and early neural connections.
- **Facial features:** Facial features such as the eyes, ears, and nose are taking shape, even though they are still fairly basic at this stage.

Week 8

- **Limb development:** The baby's limbs, which were formerly paddle-like (web-like), are now growing fingers and toes, with tiny nails beginning to form.
- **Organ development:** Major organs, including the liver, kidneys, and intestines, are rapidly forming.
- **Sensory development:** Eyes become visible and ears start to take shape.
- **Lifeline maturation:** The umbilical cord is fully developed and serves as a vital lifeline, transporting oxygen and blood to the embryo.
- **Movement:** While it's still too early for the mother to feel any movement, the baby begins to make spontaneous, reflex-like movements.

After the eighth week, healthcare providers officially refer to the embryo as a fetus, and it will remain a fetus until birth. By the end of the second month, the fetus measures about 0.5 to

1 inch in length, approximately the size of a black bean (Cleveland Clinic, 2023c).

Week 9

- **Skeleton formation:** The baby's skeleton is hardening due to a process known as ossification. Cartilage is transforming into bone.
- **External genitalia:** The external genitalia are becoming more distinct, although it may still be difficult to determine the baby's sex through ultrasound.
- **Facial features:** The face is becoming more human-like, with prominent eyelids and a more defined mouth.

Week 10

- **Muscle development:** Muscle development continues, and the baby's movements become more coordinated, but they are still too small for the mother to feel.
- **Digestive system:** The intestines are beginning to move from the umbilical cord into the abdomen. The digestive system of the baby is developing.

It's important to note that these milestones represent a general timeline, and individual growth can differ. Additionally, while many key structures are forming during this period, the risk of birth defects is relatively high, emphasizing the need for proper prenatal care and avoiding harmful substances to maintain a safe pregnancy.

6.2: Pregnancy Confirmation and Monitoring Using Blood hCG Levels

During the second month of pregnancy, the monitoring of blood hCG levels remains a crucial aspect of prenatal care. Here's a more detailed look at how hCG levels are relevant during this period.

Confirmation of Pregnancy

At two months pregnant, most women have already confirmed their pregnancy. The presence of a growing viable embryo and rising hCG levels confirms the continuation of the pregnancy.

Steady Rise of hCG Levels

- During the second month, hCG levels continue to rise, though at a slower rate than in the first few weeks of pregnancy. This hormone plays a crucial role in maintaining the corpus luteum (ovarian hormone-producing structure), which produces progesterone to sustain the pregnancy.
- While the rapid doubling seen in the early weeks may slow down, the overall trend is for hCG levels to rise gradually. These levels are still monitored to ensure the pregnancy is progressing normally.

Interpreting hCG Levels

- The specific hCG levels can vary greatly among individuals, so it is important to focus on the trends and patterns rather than absolute numbers.
- A decline in hCG levels during this stage can be alarming and may indicate a potential problem. However, it's important to note that even in healthy pregnancies, hCG levels may not regularly double at this stage as they did in the first few weeks.

Miscarriage Risk Assessment

- Monitoring hCG levels is particularly important for determining the risk of miscarriage during the second month. If there is a concern about a possible miscarriage due to symptoms such as vaginal bleeding or abdominal pain, hCG levels can provide valuable information.
- A significant drop in hCG levels, together with certain associated symptoms (vaginal spotting/bleeding, lower abdominal cramp/pain, lower back pain, and possible fever and chills), could signal an impending miscarriage. However, a single hCG measurement is inconclusive and healthcare providers often consider trends and other factors when assessing the risk (Konrad, 2007).

Ultrasound Confirmation

- In addition to blood hCG monitoring, healthcare providers may recommend an ultrasound during the second month to confirm the pregnancy's viability. An ultrasound can visualize the developing embryo or fetus, detect a heartbeat, and assess whether the pregnancy is progressing as expected.
- Ultrasound results, combined with hCG levels, provide a comprehensive picture of the pregnancy's status.

Management and Support

- If there are concerns about declining hCG levels or other signs of complications, healthcare providers will offer advice and possible interventions based on the specific situation.
- Expectant parents need emotional support and therapy during this time since facing the prospect of miscarriage can be emotionally taxing.

6.3: Miscarriages, Ectopic Pregnancy, and Multiple Gestation

Among the various pregnancy-related issues, three significant ones that require attention and understanding are miscarriages, ectopic pregnancies, and multiple gestations. Each of these conditions poses distinct risks and considerations during pregnancy. The following is a detailed explanation of these topics.

Miscarriage

A miscarriage is an unexpected event whereby a pregnancy ends prematurely before the fetus reaches viability, usually within the first 20 weeks of gestation. It can be a heartbreaking event for the expecting mom. Miscarriage is a common form of pregnancy loss. Studies suggest that about 26% of all pregnancies might experience a miscarriage, and even up to 10% of pregnancies that are clinically confirmed (Dugas & Slane, 2022).

Potential Causes and Dangers

- **Chromosomal abnormalities:** Most miscarriages in the early stages are caused by genetic or chromosomal defects in the embryo. Usually, these are serious defects that are incompatible with life.
- **Health factors:** Pre-existing medical conditions, such as diabetes or thyroid disorders, can increase the chances of miscarriage.
- **Lifestyle factors:** Smoking, alcohol usage, and certain drugs/medications can all increase the risk.

Monitoring and Prevention

- Early prenatal care and regular check-ups are essential for monitoring the pregnancy's progress and resolving any problems that may arise.
- A healthy lifestyle, including a balanced diet and avoidance of harmful substances, can help minimize the risk of miscarriage.

Ectopic Pregnancy

An ectopic pregnancy is caused by a fertilized egg attaching itself in a location other than the uterus, usually in the fallopian tube. This condition poses significant risks and necessitates prompt medical intervention. As a general rule, any unexplained lower abdominal pain/tenderness, usually on one side, with or without light vaginal bleeding, and occurring in a woman of childbearing age who may have recently experienced a missing or abnormal menstrual period is considered a medical emergency and 911 should be called right away.

Potential Causes and Dangers

- **Rupture and bleeding:** As the ectopic pregnancy progresses, the fallopian tube might burst, resulting in severe internal bleeding.
- **Life-threatening:** Ectopic pregnancies can be fatal if not treated promptly.

Monitoring and Prevention

- Early prenatal care is essential for the detection and management of ectopic pregnancies.
- When an ectopic pregnancy is diagnosed, it usually necessitates emergency medical intervention or surgery to prevent complications.

Multiple Gestation

Multiple gestation pregnancies, such as twins or triplets, present unique challenges and potential risks, especially in the early stages.

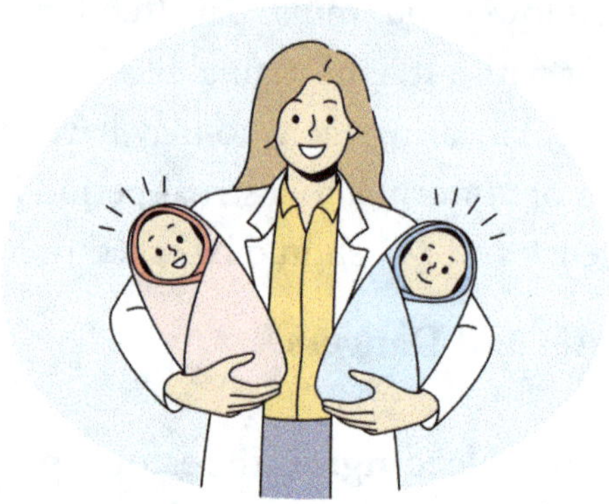

Potential Dangers and Considerations

- **Increased risks:** Multiple pregnancies are linked with a higher risk of complications such as preterm birth, low birth weight, and gestational diabetes.
- **Monitoring:** Close monitoring by healthcare personnel is essential to ensure the well-being of both the pregnant woman and the developing babies.

Management and Care

- Prenatal care for multiple gestation pregnancies often includes frequent check-ups and ultrasounds to monitor fetal development and detect any possible issues.

- To manage the high risks associated with multiple pregnancies, specialized medical treatment may be required.

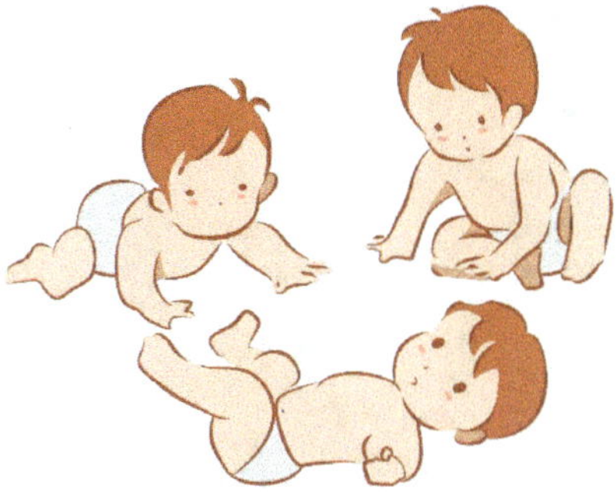

Multiple gestation

Early detection and intervention throughout the second month of pregnancy are important for addressing potential complications. Expectant mothers should contact their health-care provider with any concerns or questions. Moving on to the next chapter, transitioning into the third month marks a pivotal moment as it signals the end of the first trimester of the pregnancy journey.

Chapter 7

Pregnancy Month 3 (Weeks 11–14)

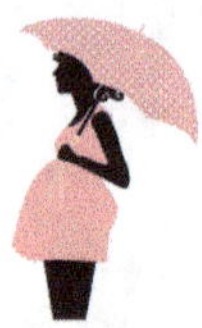

The third month of pregnancy, spanning from week 11 to 14, marks a significant milestone as it ushers in the final stretch of the first trimester. During this crucial stage, expectant mothers often experience a notable reduction in early pregnancy symptoms like nausea and fatigue, while the fetus undergoes remarkable growth and development. This stage is distinguished by thrilling milestones like the baby's rapidly developing organs, recognizable facial features, and the possibility of hearing the baby's heartbeat.

7.1: Your Baby's Developmental Milestones in the Third Month

During the 3rd month of pregnancy, your baby undergoes significant developmental milestones as they continue to grow and develop within the womb. Here are the developmental milestones for each week during this period.

Week 11

- The fingers and toes of your baby begin to separate.
- The baby's facial features become clearer, particularly the formation of the nose and mouth.
- They can produce subtle, reflexive movements, although they're too tiny for you to feel.

Week 12

- Your baby's body starts producing urine, which is discharged into the amniotic fluid.
- The baby's skin is very thin and blood vessels can be seen.
- Their brain continues to grow rapidly, with billions of neurons being formed.
- The placenta is fully formed and assumes the role of providing oxygen and nutrients to the baby (Cleveland Clinic, 2022d).

Week 13

- The digestive system of your baby is developing, and the intestines begin to move into the abdomen from the umbilical cord.
- The baby begins to develop vocal cords, although they won't be used for speech until much later.
- Fine hair, known as lanugo, covers the skin to help regulate body temperature.

Week 14

- They can make sucking motions with their mouth and may even be able to suck their thumb.
- Limb movements become better coordinated, and they may begin to make small, purposeful movements.
- It's important to keep in mind that each baby develops at their own pace, and these are just estimates. Regular prenatal check-ups with your healthcare provider can help ensure that your baby is developing properly.

7.2: What to Expect This Month

The third month of pregnancy marks the end of the first trimester. Here's what you can generally expect during this stage of pregnancy.

Physical Changes for the Mother

- **Morning sickness:** While some women may still experience morning sickness, it usually begins to improve by the end of the third month.
- **Breast changes:** Your breasts may become more sensitive and increase in size. Additionally, your areolas may darken and veins may become more prominent.
- **Fatigue:** You may still feel fatigued and require extra rest throughout this trimester, but some women begin to regain energy.

- **Weight gain:** You may have gained a few pounds by this point, but weight gain is typically moderate in the first trimester.

Fetal Development

- **Fetal size:** By the end of the third month, the fetus is about three-and-a-half inches long and weighs around an ounce and a half (*Embryonic & fetal development*, 2015). It is roughly the size of a lemon.
- **Organs and systems:** The development of key organs and systems such as the heart, kidneys, and the digestive system continues. Fingernails and toenails begin to grow.
- **Sexual differentiation:** In some cases, it may be possible to detect the baby's sex through ultrasound near the end of this trimester, but it is more reliably determined later in the pregnancy.

Prenatal Care

- **Prenatal check-ups:** Regular prenatal visits to your healthcare provider are essential during this period. Another ultrasound may be performed to monitor the baby's development and health.
- **Genetic testing:** Some genetic tests, such as the first-trimester screening or the cell-free DNA test, might be offered to determine the risk of certain genetic conditions.

Emotional Changes

- **Emotional rollercoaster:** Pregnancy hormones can cause mood swings, so it is a good idea to communicate your feelings with your partner and healthcare provider.
- **Bonding:** As the pregnancy progresses, many expectant mothers often begin to develop a stronger emotional bond with their unborn child.

Diet and Nutrition

Focus on a balanced diet that includes folate-rich foods. Continue taking prenatal vitamins and supplements as directed by your healthcare professional to address particular nutritional needs during this crucial stage.

Exercise

- **Moderate activity:** Moderate activity is generally safe and recommended during pregnancy. Discuss your workout program with your healthcare provider to ensure it's suitable for your specific situation.

Safety Considerations

- **Avoid toxins:** Continue to avoid exposure to harmful substances like alcohol, tobacco, and certain medications.
- **Safety precautions:** It is important to take precautions to prevent falls or accidents that could harm you or your developing baby.

Keep in mind that every pregnancy is unique, and some women may experience different symptoms and developments during this stage. Maintaining open communication with your healthcare professional and following their advice is essential for a healthy and safe pregnancy.

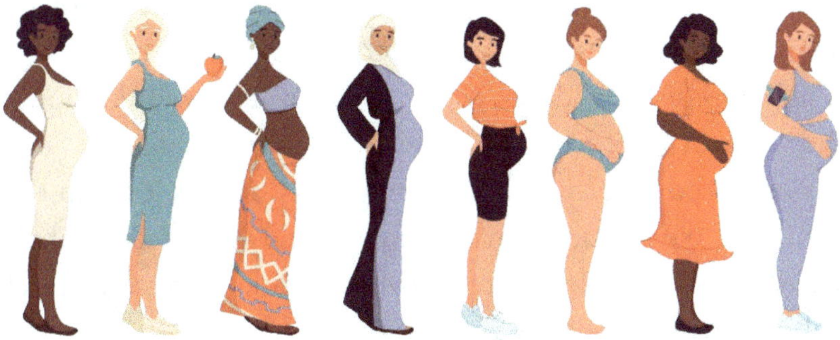

Every pregnancy is unique

7.3: High Risk Moms

High-risk mothers are pregnant women who have a higher chance of having a baby with neural tube defects (NTDs) or genetic abnormalities due to a range of factors, including a family history of NTDs, certain medications, or medical conditions such as diabetes. High-risk moms require closer monitoring during pregnancy.

1st vaginal ultrasound: High-risk pregnant women typically undergo their first prenatal screening through a vaginal ultrasound. This screening is usually conducted during the early weeks of pregnancy, specifically between weeks 10 and 14 (Lee et al., 2023). Ultrasound is a safe and noninvasive procedure that enables healthcare providers to observe the developing fetus. During the ultrasound, the healthcare provider carefully examines the fetal anatomy, with a special focus on neural tube development, searching for any abnormalities or defects that could be an early indicator of NTDs.

Moms not considered high risk: Pregnant women who are not at high risk for neural tube defects are also screened, but their testing schedule is different. Low-risk moms are routinely screened for NTDs between weeks 12–15 of their pregnancy. This screening is done using a blood test called Alpha-Fetoprotein (AFP) level, instead of an ultrasound. AFP is a protein produced by the developing fetus, and its levels in the mother's blood can provide information about the baby's health. If the AFP levels are elevated, it could indicate a neural tube defect (Darouich et al., 2015).

7.4: What Are NTDs?

Neural tube defects (NTDs) are a set of innate abnormalities that hinder the proper formation of the brain, spinal cord, or their protective layers. These defects manifest in the initial stages of fetal development, characterized by an incomplete closure of the neural tube—the precursor to the brain and spinal cord. NTDs can lead to significant health issues and life-long disabilities for the affected child.

Causes

The causes of NTDs are not always clear, but several factors can contribute to their development.

- **Genetics:** NTDs can run in families, implying a genetic component. Certain gene mutations or variations may raise a baby's risk of having an NTD.

- **Environmental factors:** Some environmental factors during pregnancy, such as insufficient intake of folic acid (a B vitamin), exposure to certain medications, and maternal obesity, may raise the incidence of NTDs.
- **Folic acid deficiency:** A lack of folic acid before and during early pregnancy is a well-established risk factor for NTDs. Folic acid is required for healthy neural tube formation and women of reproductive age are urged to take folic acid supplements to lessen the risk.

Diagnostic Methods

- **Prenatal screening:** Doctors may offer prenatal screening tests to determine the risk of NTDs during pregnancy. Maternal serum alpha-fetoprotein (MSAFP) screening is one of these tests, which analyzes a specific protein in the mother's blood. MSAFP levels that are elevated may suggest a higher risk.
- **Prenatal imaging:** Some NTDs can be detected with ultrasound scanning during pregnancy. Ultrasound images may reveal disorders such as spina bifida.
- **Amniocentesis:** In certain cases, doctors may suggest performing amniocentesis, a procedure that involves extracting a sample of amniotic fluid and examining it for any genetic abnormalities. This is usually recommended when other screening tests or risk factors indicate a high likelihood of complications.

Prevention in Pregnancy

To prevent NTDs during pregnancy, it is important to reduce risk factors and ensure adequate nutrition.

- **Folic acid supplementation:** Women of childbearing age are recommended to take a daily folic acid supplement of 400 micrograms before and during early pregnancy (CDC, 2022). This has the potential to greatly minimize the risk of NTDs.
- **Healthy lifestyle:** Maintaining a healthy weight, avoiding smoking and drinking alcohol, and managing any chronic health conditions are essential during pregnancy to reduce the risk of NTDs.
- **Genetic counseling:** This can be helpful for prospective parents with a family history of NTDs or other risk factors. It can assist them in understanding their risk and making informed decisions.
- **Medication review:** It is important for pregnant women to consult with their healthcare provider regarding any medication they are taking, as some drugs may increase the risk of NTDs.
- **Prenatal care:** Regular prenatal check-ups and screenings are crucial to monitor the development of the baby and to detect any potential issues that may require medical attention.

Moving on from the first to the second trimester marks changes in both physical and emotional experiences, setting the stage for the next chapter, which will look at body changes, baby development, and mood shifts during this transformative period.

Second Trimester Overview

A mother's joy begins when new life is stirring inside; when a tiny heartbeat is heard for the first time, and a playful kick reminds her that she is never alone.

— Unknown

The second trimester of pregnancy is commonly referred to as the "honeymoon" phase because many women begin to feel better during this time compared to the first trimester. Here's an overview of some key aspects of the second trimester:

- **Feeling better:** Many women experience relief from the morning sickness and fatigue, which are prevalent throughout the first trimester. The second trimester is often linked with increased energy and a general sense of well-being.

- **Pregnancy glow:** The so-called "pregnancy glow" is a phenomenon in which some women appear to have healthier, more radiant skin during pregnancy. It is thought to be related to increased blood flow and hormonal changes. While it is not guaranteed for everyone, some women do experience clearer skin and a certain radiance.
- **Announcing pregnancy:** Many women prefer to wait until after the first trimester to announce their pregnancy because the risk of miscarriage drops dramatically after this time. It is a personal choice and often depends on individual circumstances.
- **Doubling numbers:** This refers to the measurement of hCG hormone levels in the blood. In a healthy pregnancy, hCG levels should roughly double every 48 to 72 hours. Consistent doubling of hCG levels is a positive sign of a developing pregnancy.
- **Eating for two:** While you're not eating for two, it's vital to maintain a healthy diet during pregnancy to ensure that you and your baby get the nutrients they need. Weight management is also needed during this trimester to promote healthy weight gain.

Second-Trimester Concerns

- **Heartburn:** Hormonal changes can cause the esophageal sphincter to relax, resulting in heartburn. It can be managed with dietary changes and over-the-counter antacids.

- **Stretch marks:** Stretch marks appear in many women as their skin stretches to accommodate the growing baby. Moisturizers can help reduce their appearance.
- **Sexual activity:** While generally safe throughout the second trimester, consult with your healthcare provider for specific advice based on your pregnancy.

Vaginal bleeding during the second trimester of pregnancy can be caused by a variety of factors, such as late-onset abortion, placenta previa, placental abruption, cervical changes, or infections. The severity of the bleeding is determined by the cause, but it should always be taken seriously. If you experience vaginal bleeding during the second trimester, contact your healthcare professional immediately to assess the situation.

Fetal Movements

- **Fluttering:** Fetal movements, also described as fluttering or gentle taps, can start as early as the second trimester, usually around the 18th to 20th week.
- **Monitoring fetal movements:** Kick counting is frequently recommended by healthcare experts as a method of monitoring fetal movements. You should feel a certain number of movements within a specified time frame daily.
- **Second vs. third trimester:** Fetal movements become stronger and more pronounced as pregnancy advances, particularly in the third trimester.

- **Activities associated with increased movements:** Eating, drinking something cold or sweet, or sleeping on your left side can all cause fetal movements.
- **Normal decrease:** It's normal for fetal movements to decrease when the fetus is sleeping or as the pregnancy advances because the baby has less room to move. However, if you notice a significant and sudden decrease, contact your healthcare provider.
- **Gender determination:** Many parents-to-be opt for an ultrasound during the second trimester to discover the baby's gender.

Remember that every pregnancy is different, and it is essential to consult with your healthcare provider for personalized guidance and to address any specific concerns or issues you may have at this time.

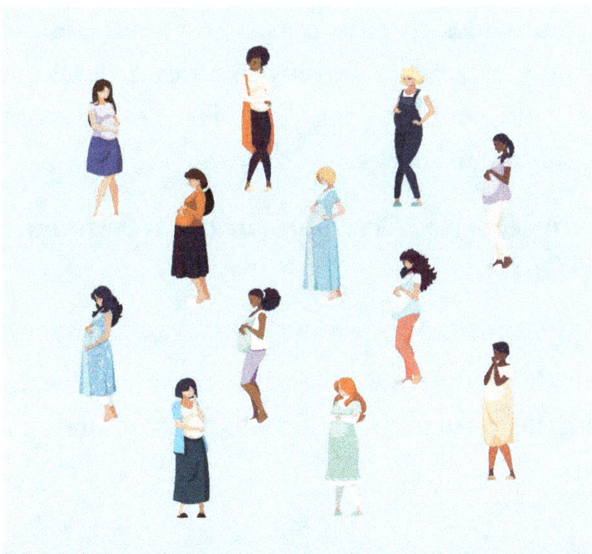

Chapter 8

Pregnancy Month 4 (Weeks 15–18)

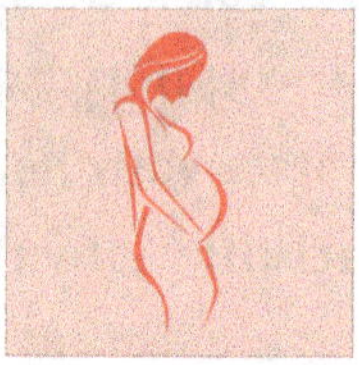

You are now in your fourth month of pregnancy, spanning from weeks 15 to 18. It is essential to focus on maintaining a balanced and nutritious diet. Discuss any dietary concerns or specific recommendations with your healthcare provider to ensure a healthy and safe pregnancy. You will now experience various significant developments in your body and your growing baby. Here is a list of what to expect in this crucial period.

8.1: Your Baby's Developmental Milestones in the Fourth Month

During the fourth month of pregnancy, your baby undergoes significant developmental milestones in terms of size, appearance, and the formation of key body structures. Here's an overview.

- **Size:** As your pregnancy progresses into the fourth month, you may begin to feel more connected to your baby as you experience their movements and witness their development during prenatal check-ups and ultrasounds. By the end of the fourth month, your baby is approximately six inches long and weighs around four ounces (American Pregnancy Association, n.d.).

- **Appearance:** Your baby's appearance gets more human-like and less tadpole-like at this stage. The head, body, and limbs may all be identified, and facial characteristics become more defined. Your baby's eyes, ears, and nose continue to develop, and their facial expressions may become apparent on ultrasound scans.

Developing Structures

- **Nervous system:** During the fourth month, the neurological system is quickly developing. Your baby's brain is developing, and neural connections are emerging, allowing them to perform numerous sensory and motor skills.
- **Musculoskeletal system:** Muscles and bones are still growing. Your baby's limbs can move and you may notice mild fluttering movements, though they are not yet powerful enough to be felt from the outside.
- **Digestive system:** The baby's digestive system continues to mature as the intestines expand further and intricate organs, such as the stomach, begin to take shape within the developing abdomen.
- **Reproductive system:** If you're expecting a male baby, the prostate gland and external genitalia are

developing. For female babies, the ovaries contain millions of eggs, and the uterus is forming.

- **Sensory organs:** Taste buds are developing on your baby's tongue, and they are beginning to make sucking motions. Although the eyelids remain closed, your baby's eyes may begin to move beneath them, and they may be able to detect light.
- **Skin:** Your baby's skin is still thin and transparent, but it is thickening and developing layers.
- **Umbilical cord:** The umbilical cord continues to deliver essential nutrients and oxygen to your baby while also removing waste products.

8.2: What to Expect This Month

Several physical and emotional changes can be expected throughout the fourth month of pregnancy, which spans from the beginning of week 15 to the end of week 18.

Physical Changes

- **Baby bump:** Your tummy will continue to grow, and by the end of the fourth month, you may start to show a noticeable baby bump.
- **Weight gain:** You will likely experience gradual weight gain. Your healthcare provider can advise you on the proper rate of weight gain for your specific situation.
- **Breast changes:** Your breasts may continue to enlarge and become more tender. You may also notice the darkening of the areolas and the formation

of tiny bumps (Montgomery's tubercles) on the areolas.

- **Skin changes:** Some women may experience changes in their skin, including the appearance of stretch marks or a dark line down the center of the abdomen (linea nigra). Your skin may become more sensitive as well.
- **Hair and nails:** Hormonal changes can result in changes in hair and nail growth. Some women develop thicker, shinier hair, while others may experience hair thinning.
- **Increased energy:** Many women report having more energy in this month than in the previous months when morning sickness and fatigue are common. You may begin to feel more like yourself and be able to resume some of your regular activities.

Emotional Changes

- **Emotional rollercoaster:** Pregnancy hormones can cause mood swings, so you might be going through a range of emotions, from joy and excitement to moments of anxiety or despair. This is both natural and to be expected.
- **Bonding:** As your baby's movements become more noticeable, you may begin to develop a stronger bond with your baby, strengthening your emotional connection.
- **Anticipation:** As your pregnancy advances, you and your partner may begin to feel a growing sense of

anticipation and excitement about the arrival of your baby.

Medical Appointments

- Regular prenatal check-ups with your healthcare practitioner may be recommended to monitor your health and the growth of your baby.
- In the fourth month, some women have an ultrasound, which can reveal important details about the baby's health and gender if you choose to find out.
- During this trimester, your healthcare professional may discuss the many prenatal testing and screenings available.

8.3 Begin Developing Your Birth Plan

A birth plan is a written document that outlines your preferences and expectations for the childbirth process. It is important to remember that labor and delivery can be unpredictable, but having a birth plan will help you communicate your objectives to your healthcare team and ensure that your choices are considered as much as possible. Although birth plans are implemented in the third trimester, it is recommended to begin gathering information and developing your birth plan during the second trimester so that you have sufficient time and energy to establish your goal for every aspect of the labor and delivery process by the time the third trimester rolls by. Below are steps to guide you to begin developing your unique birth plan during this second trimester.

Research and Gather Information

When preparing for childbirth, it is important to educate yourself on the different phases of labor and delivery. Various resources are available for educating yourself on the phases of labor and delivery, including

- childbirth classes, published books, and trustworthy online sources.
- learning about labor stages, pain management options, and available delivery interventions can assist with developing a well-informed birth plan.

Consult Your Healthcare Provider

Discuss your pregnancy and birth plans with your healthcare provider. They can provide valuable advice, address any concerns, and help you understand any medical conditions or circumstances that may impact your birth plan.

Personal Preferences

Personal preferences will influence decisions about factors such as pain management, labor positions, and who you want to have with you during the delivery process. Here are some things to consider:

- Do you prefer a natural delivery with minimal medical interventions or are you open to accepting interventions if they become necessary?
- What kind of pain relief options are you interested in? Options include epidurals, nitrous oxide, or

natural pain management strategies like breathing exercises and movement.

- Do you have a specific location in mind for giving birth? This could be at home, in a birthing center, or in a hospital setting.
- Do you want your partner, family members, or a doula to be part of your birthing support team?

Labor and Delivery Environment

You should research the different labor and delivery options available in your area and weigh the pros and cons of each. Your preferences should also be discussed with your healthcare provider to ensure that they align with your medical needs.

Medical Interventions and Procedures

You should also educate yourself on common medical procedures and interventions, such as episiotomies, vacuum extraction, and cesarean sections. Talk with your healthcare provider about whether these are necessary and how you would like them to be handled.

Pain Management

Don't forget to include your pain management preferences in your birth plan. There are numerous pain management options available, such as

- **Natural techniques:** Exploring natural childbirth techniques such as hypnobirthing, Bradley, Lamaze, and Alexander methods, along with options like water delivery, can help you manage pain and anxiety during labor by focusing on relaxation, controlled breathing, and supportive birthing practices (American Pregnancy Association, n.d.-d). Water birth involves laboring and occasionally delivering in a warm water tub, which can offer pain relief and comfort.

- **Epidural:** An epidural is a regional anesthesia option that provides pain relief from the waist down. It is injected into the spine through a catheter and can provide effective pain relief during labor and delivery.
- **IV medications:** Intravenous medications, such as opioids, can be administered to provide temporary pain relief. They can help alleviate pain but may have side effects such as drowsiness.
- **Nitrous oxide (laughing gas):** Some hospitals offer nitrous oxide, which can be inhaled to help control pain and anxiety during childbirth. It is a self-administered option that provides mild pain relief.
- **Sterile water injections:** To reduce back pain during labor, sterile water injections can be given in the lower back. This procedure is less prevalent; however, it may be offered in some healthcare facilities.
- **Transcutaneous electrical nerve stimulation (TENS):** TENS machines deliver mild electrical impulses to the skin, which can assist in relieving pain by interfering with pain signals. It's often used to treat back pain during early labor.
- **Acupressure and massage:** Trained professionals can employ acupressure and massage techniques to provide pain relief and relaxation during childbirth.

- **Spinal block:** A spinal block, like an epidural, is a type of regional anesthesia that provides pain relief for procedures like Cesarean section.

Labor Positions and Movement

It's important to consider the labor positions and movements that make you feel most comfortable. These preferences should be included in your birth plan, as certain postures can help alleviate discomfort and facilitate a smoother labor process.

Postpartum and Infant Care

It is also recommended to include your postpartum and infant care preferences, such as immediate skin-to-skin contact with your baby, delayed cord clamping, and nursing of your baby. Your choices should be clearly stated in your birth plan.

Emergency Situations

Additionally, discuss emergency situations with your healthcare professional and prepare a contingency plan. Be sure to include your preferences for emergency response, such as who should be consulted and what interventions are considered acceptable.

Writing Your Birth Plan

Creating a birth plan involves gathering and documenting your preferences and options in a straightforward way. It is important to keep it basic and easy to understand. Share this plan with your healthcare provider so that they are aware of your preferences and can incorporate them into your care plan.

It is important to note that during labor and delivery, flexibility is crucial. While birth plans serve as a guide, unforeseen complications may arise, necessitating immediate medical decisions. Open communication with your healthcare team is important to achieving the best possible outcome for both you and your baby. As your pregnancy progresses, your healthcare professional can assist you in refining and finalizing your birth plan.

During the fourth month of pregnancy, experiences can vary, so it is important to stay in touch with your healthcare provider for a safe pregnancy. As the fifth month starts, your baby's development and your own experiences will continue to evolve, with new milestones, physical changes, and growing anticipation for your baby's arrival.

Chapter 9

Pregnancy Month 5 (Weeks 19–22)

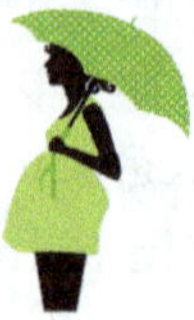

The fifth month of pregnancy marks a critical turning point in the lives of expectant moms. Many women have noticed a reduction in morning sickness and fatigue by this time and they begin to feel more energized and comfortable. During this month, the baby's development becomes more obvious, with the mother frequently feeling the first fluttering movements as the fetus grows and matures.

9.1: Your Baby's Developmental Milestones in the Fifth Month

Your baby will reach key developmental milestones in the fifth month of pregnancy, which will contribute to their growth and readiness for life outside the womb. This period spans from week 19 to week 22, and during this time, your baby's growth, appearance, developing structures, and first fetal movements all change dramatically.

- **Size and appearance:** By the end of the fifth month, your baby can have a length of approximately 9 to 10 inches and weigh around one pound (Cleveland Clinic, 2023c). This substantial growth reflects their increasing maturity and readiness for the outside world.
- **Fetal movements:** At around week 19, your baby's muscles are strengthening, and most women begin to feel the first sensations of their baby's movements, such as kicks and punches. This is known as "quickening" and is a momentous milestone for expectant mothers, as it provides a tangible connection to their growing baby.
- **Unique fingerprints:** By this stage, your baby has developed its own unique set of fingerprints, signaling the start of their individuality.
- **Sensory brain development:** Around week 20, your baby's brain begins to develop the area responsible for processing the five senses. This lays the foundation for your baby's ability to see, hear, taste, smell, and touch after birth.
- **Nail growth:** Your baby's nail growth extends to the tips of their fingers.
- **Bone marrow and blood cell production:** By week 21, your baby's bone marrow is functioning, helping to produce blood cells, which are needed for oxygen transport and overall health.
- **Improved coordination:** During week 21, your baby's limb movements become more coordinated and frequent, emphasizing the development of their motor skills.

- **Sensory development:** By week 22, your baby can hear your heartbeat, the rumbling of your stomach, and your breathing. This sensory connection with the external world is a crucial part of their development.
- **Lanugo hair and vernix caseosa:** Throughout this month, your baby's body continues to be covered with fine hair called lanugo. Additionally, a protective substance called vernix caseosa forms a layer on the skin, protecting it from the amniotic fluid. Both of these features are temporary and will be shed before birth.
- **Eyebrows and eyelashes:** By week 22, your baby's facial features become more prominent, with the appearance of eyebrows and eyelashes.
- **Meconium formation:** During this period, our baby's first bowel movement, meconium, is produced in the intestinal tract. Meconium is typically dark and sticky, and the newborn passes it quickly after delivery.
- **Heartbeat audible:** At week 22, you can use a stethoscope to hear your baby's heartbeat, providing an auditory connection to your developing child.

It's important to note that these milestones are general guidelines and can vary from one pregnancy to another. Some babies will achieve certain developmental stages earlier than others. Regular prenatal visits with your healthcare practitioner are essential for monitoring your baby's growth and ensuring that they are developing normally.

9.2: What to Expect This Month

During the fifth month of pregnancy, there are several key developments and changes that both the expectant mother and the developing fetus will experience. These changes can be monitored and evaluated through various measurements, including belly measurements in centimeters (fundal height) and landmark measurements beginning from 20 weeks.

Belly Measurements (Fundal Height)

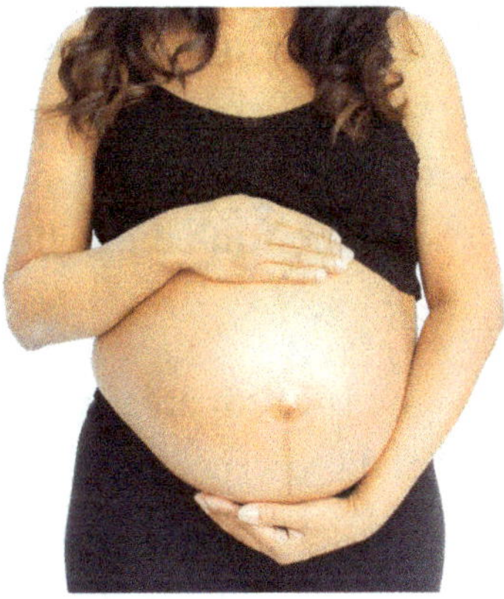

Fundal height

Fundal height is a common measurement taken during prenatal check-ups to determine the growth and development of the fetus. It involves measuring the distance from the pubic bone to the top of the uterus (fundus) using a measuring tape. Fundal height is usually measured in centimeters, and it roughly corresponds to the number of weeks of gestation (Cleveland Clinic, 2022). This measurement assists healthcare providers to monitor the baby's growth and detect any potential problems, such as fetal growth restriction or excessive growth.

During the fifth month (19–22 weeks) of pregnancy, the fundal height will steadily increase as the baby grows. The measurement can provide useful information about the baby's growth rate and whether it is consistent with the expected gestational age.

At around 20 weeks, the fundal height should be approximately at the level of the navel (belly button), though there can be slight variations among individuals (Cleveland Clinic, 2022). As pregnancy progresses, the fundal height tends to increase gradually. Since it closely aligns with the gestational week count, at 22 weeks, the fundal height might be around 22 centimeters.

Measuring fundal height is a valuable method for healthcare providers to monitor fetal growth. If you're informed that the fetus's measurements deviate from the expected schedule, don't be overly concerned. Typically, this indicates the need for additional tests or an ultrasound. In most cases, the fetus is developing normally. If you have any worries about your fundal height or the fetus's size, it's advisable to discuss them with your healthcare provider.

Landmark Measurements Beginning From 20 Weeks

A 20-week ultrasound scan, often known as the anatomy scan or mid-pregnancy ultrasound, is conducted to ensure the baby's healthy development. Some of the landmark measurements taken during this ultrasound include

- **Fetal length (crown-rump length):** This is measured from the top of the baby's head (crown) to the bottom of the spine (rump). It estimates the size and gestational age of the fetus.
- **Head circumference:** Measuring the circumference of the baby's head allows you to assess the development of the brain and skull. It is a key sign of the baby's overall health.
- **Abdominal circumference:** The measurement of the baby's abdominal circumference aids in determining the growth of the belly and its organs.
- **Femur length:** This measurement is used to determine the length of the baby's thigh bone (femur) and offers information about the baby's limb development.
- **Levels of amniotic fluid:** The measurement of amniotic fluid surrounding the baby is crucial, as an elevated level might indicate potential problems. While it is essential to note that normal amniotic fluid levels can fluctuate throughout pregnancy, maintaining an adequate amount is vital for proper fetal development and movement. Healthcare providers will monitor and assess amniotic fluid levels during routine ultrasounds.
- **Placental position:** The position and condition of the placenta are assessed. A healthy placenta is essential for supplying nutrition and oxygen to the fetus. The location of the placenta can vary, but it is normally attached to the uterine wall away from the cervix. However, if the placenta is too close to or

covering the cervix (placenta previa), it may require monitoring and possible interventions.

- **Fetal organs:** The ultrasound may also be used to inspect the baby's internal organs, such as the heart, kidneys, and bladder, to identify any abnormalities or developmental concerns. Normal measurements for specific organs can vary widely and depend on gestational age.

These landmark measurements and assessments are essential for monitoring the well-being and growth of the fetus, identifying any potential anomalies, and providing necessary medical interventions or support if needed.

Fetal Biometry: What's Normal and When to Be Concerned

This is a routine measurement that shows whether the fetus is measuring smaller or larger than normal for its age. It is like a measuring tape for your developing baby during pregnancy and helps doctors monitor your baby's growth. However, what's considered "normal" varies and depends on several factors. Each baby has its own unique path of growth and healthcare providers take into account a variety of factors when analyzing these measurements.

Normal fetal biometry ranges differ depending on factors such as gestational age and individual pregnancy characteristics. At roughly 20 weeks gestation, the average measurements are 17.5cm for the head circumference (HC), 14.9cm for the abdominal circumference (AC), 4.9cm for the biparietal diameter (BPD), and 3.2cm for the femur length (FL) (Cleveland Clinic, 2023h).

These numbers are useful, but they're not the whole story. You will also receive "percentile" values, comparing your baby's size to others of the same age. For example, if your baby's abdominal circumference is in the 75th percentile, they are larger than most babies their age. But don't worry, it doesn't always indicate trouble. Healthcare providers usually worry when measurements fall below the 10th percentile or above the 90th percentile.

Understanding Abnormal Results

If your fetal biometry results seem unusual, your healthcare provider may recommend more ultrasounds. These additional scans aid in tracking your baby's growth over time and detecting any changes. They may also examine your blood test and urinalysis results to gain further insight into what is going on.

Here is what abnormal fetal biometry results could suggest:

- A smaller-than-average measurement may be an indication of fetal growth issues or placental problems.
- A larger-than-average measurement might suggest gestational diabetes in the birth parent.

Remember, slight variations are common and most babies grow up healthily within a normal size and weight range. Don't be alarmed if one ultrasound yields unexpected results.

Trust your healthcare provider to guide you through the next steps.

9.3: Sleep Hygiene

Sleep Positions: Finding the Right One

As your tummy grows, sleeping positions can become a challenge. The ideal position for most pregnant women during this stage is to sleep on their left side. This position enhances blood circulation to the fetus and reduces the pressure on key blood vessels like the vena cava, which can get compressed when lying on your back.

Use Pillows for Support

Pillows are your true pals during pregnancy. Consider using a pregnancy pillow or a combination of regular pillows to support your developing belly and reduce pressure on your back. For extra comfort, place one pillow between your knees, another under your belly, and one behind your back.

Elevate Your Upper Body

If you're suffering from heartburn or acid reflux, consider raising your upper body slightly by supporting your upper torso with pillows. This can reduce discomfort by preventing stomach acid from flowing back into your esophagus.

Stay Hydrated, but Time It Right

Staying hydrated is essential, but limit your fluid intake in the evening to reduce nighttime bathroom trips. Dehydration can cause discomfort, but avoiding excessive liquids before bedtime will help you sleep better.

Create a Relaxing Bedtime Routine

Establish a relaxing bedtime routine to communicate to your body that it's time to unwind. This might include relaxing activities such as reading a book, taking a warm bath, or practicing gentle prenatal yoga or stretching exercises for muscle relaxation.

Manage Stress and Anxiety

Pregnancy can generate worries and anxieties. Consider practicing relaxation techniques, such as deep breathing exercises or meditation, before going to bed to relieve stress.

Maintain a Comfortable Sleep Environment

Ensure your bedroom is conducive to sleep. Maintain a dark, cool, and quiet environment. To improve your sleep quality, invest in a comfortable mattress and bedding.

Nap Smartly

Short naps during the day can help combat fatigue, but avoid resting too close to bedtime because it may disrupt your nighttime sleep. If necessary, take a short nap early in the day.

Communicate With Your Partner

If you share a bed with a partner, communicate your needs. They can be helpful by adjusting their sleep position or being understanding of your changing sleep patterns.

Consult Your Healthcare Provider

If sleep problems persist or become serious, don't hesitate to consult your healthcare provider. They can offer personalized advice and address any specific concerns or medical conditions that may be interfering with your sleep.

As the fifth month of pregnancy comes to an end, the excitement for what lies ahead grows stronger. Your body changes dramatically with each passing day and your baby's growth continues to unfold. Turn the page and enter the sixth month, where new milestones and experiences await on this incredible journey to motherhood.

Chapter 10

Pregnancy Month 6 (Weeks 23–26)

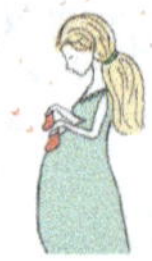

The sixth month of pregnancy is a period of rapid growth for the baby as key organs like the lungs, brain, and eyes continue to develop. To support this growth, it is essential for moms to follow dietary guidelines recommended by their healthcare provider.

10.1: Your Baby's Developmental Milestones in the Sixth Month

During the sixth month, significant progress is made in lung development, sensory awareness, and fat accumulation. Details of the developmental milestones for this month are provided below.

- **Fetal size and weight gain:** During this period, your baby's weight gain accelerates rapidly. By the end of the sixth month, the baby is approximately 12 inches long and weighs about two pounds. It continues to mature, accumulate body fat, and respond to stimuli like sound and light (Cleveland Clinic, 2023c).

- **Lung development:** The lungs reach a crucial phase where gas exchange sacs begin to form, enhancing their functionality.
- **Audible heartbeat:** The baby's heartbeat can be heard using a stethoscope.
- **Chance of survival:** Around 23–24 weeks, there is a chance of survival with intensive care if premature birth occurs.
- **Surfactant production:** Between weeks 25 and 26, the lungs continue to expand, and lung cells begin to produce surfactant, which helps keep the lungs open between breaths after birth.
- **Fat accumulation:** Fat progressively accumulates beneath the baby's skin, making it less wrinkled and plumper.
- **Rapid eye movements:** Ultrasound scans can now identify rapid eye movements, indicating brain development (*Embryonic & fetal development*, 2015).
- **Sensory development:** The baby's senses continue to grow, with the ability to suck on fingers or hands and react to loud noises.
- **Skin and eye pigmentation:** Melanin production begins, determining skin and eye color.
- **Fully developed lungs:** By week 26, the baby's lungs are fully formed but not yet suitable for external respiration.
- **Amniotic fluid changes:** The amniotic fluid starts to diminish as the pregnancy progresses.

10.2: What to Expect This Month

The sixth month of pregnancy marks the latter part of the second trimester, and it's a crucial stage as the baby continues to grow and develop, setting the stage for the final trimester and birth. Here are some key changes that you can expect during this time:

- **Visible baby bump:** Your baby bump will be pretty visible by the end of the sixth month, and you may have gained some weight. Your belly will continue to grow, and you may need to start wearing maternity clothing for comfort.
- **Increased energy:** Many women notice an increase in energy throughout the second trimester, making this month more enjoyable than the first month when fatigue was common.
- **Reduced morning sickness:** Morning sickness and nausea, which are prevalent in the first trimester, often begin to fade throughout the second trimester, helping you feel better overall.
- **Fetal movements:** You will most likely be more aware of your baby's movements. These movements might range from light flutters to stronger kicks and rolls. Feeling your baby move can form a strong emotional bond between you and your baby.
- **Glowing skin and hair:** Hormonal changes cause some women to have better skin and hair during pregnancy. However, others may still face skin issues or hair changes, as every pregnant woman is affected differently.

- **Increased appetite:** During this month, your hunger may increase. A healthy diet is necessary for providing essential nutrients to you and your growing baby.
- **Regular prenatal checkups:** You will continue to have regular prenatal checkups with your healthcare provider. These visits are crucial for monitoring your baby's development and addressing any concerns or queries you may have.
- **Weight gain:** You can expect to gain weight throughout pregnancy, and your healthcare provider will keep an eye on this to ensure it is within a healthy range. The amount of weight you should gain depends on various factors, including your pre-pregnancy weight.
- **Heartburn and indigestion:** As the uterus grows and puts pressure on the stomach, some women may experience heartburn and indigestion.
- **Emotional changes:** Hormonal fluctuations can have an impact on your mood. During the second trimester, some women feel more emotionally stable, while others may experience mood swings.
- **Preparing for the baby:** Now is a great time to start thinking about baby names, nursery decor, and childbirth classes. It's also a wonderful time to talk about your birth plans with your doctor.
- **Swelling and minor discomfort:** It is normal to experience some swelling in your feet, ankles, and hands, but if it gets severe or is accompanied by other troubling symptoms like high blood pressure, you should contact your healthcare provider.

- **Braxton-Hicks contractions:** Some women may begin to experience Braxton-Hicks contractions, which are practice contractions that help prepare the uterus for labor. They are usually mild and irregular.
- **Nesting instinct:** Some women may have a "nesting instinct," where they have a strong urge to clean, organize, and prepare for the baby's arrival. This is a normal part of the nesting process.

Remember that each pregnancy is unique, and symptoms and experiences may differ from one individual to the next. During this important time in your life, it is crucial to be in constant touch with your healthcare provider, follow their suggestions, and prioritize self-care. If you have any concerns or notice any strange symptoms, please consult them for advice and reassurance.

10.3: Some Second Trimester Medical Problems to Watch For

There are various medical concerns that healthcare providers may monitor and handle throughout the second trimester of pregnancy. Here's a rundown of some of these issues:

Gestational Diabetes

- **Definition:** Gestational diabetes is a type of diabetes that occurs during pregnancy when the body's insulin production is insufficient to meet the increasing demands.
- **Implications during pregnancy:** It can cause complications for both the mother and baby if not

properly treated. High blood sugar levels may enhance the risk of having a large baby, preterm birth, and preeclampsia.
- **Implications after pregnancy:** Most women with gestational diabetes return to normal blood sugar levels after giving birth. However, they are at a higher risk of developing type 2 diabetes later in life and should be monitored regularly.

Oral Glucose Tolerance Test (OGTT)

- **Definition:** OGTT is a pregnancy diagnostic test used to assess if a pregnant woman has gestational diabetes.
- **Procedure:** It involves fasting overnight, followed by the consumption of a sugary solution (glucose drink). To evaluate blood sugar levels, blood samples are taken at particular intervals (usually before consuming the glucose solution and again one and two hours afterward) (NIH, 2020).
- **Diagnosis**: Elevated blood sugar levels one or two hours after drinking the glucose drink may indicate gestational diabetes.

The OGTT is an important aspect of the gestational diabetes assessment because it helps healthcare providers identify and manage the condition in pregnant women. If gestational diabetes is detected by the OGTT, it can be controlled with dietary changes, lifestyle adjustments, and, in some situations, medication to control blood sugar levels and limit the potential dangers faced by both the mother and the baby.

Glucose Resistance

- **Definition:** Glucose resistance, or insulin resistance, occurs when the body's cells do not give a proper response to insulin. This can cause high blood glucose levels.
- **Implications during pregnancy:** It is often a precursor to gestational diabetes and, if untreated, can lead to similar problems. Insulin resistance in pregnancy may necessitate further monitoring and dietary adjustments.
- **Implications after pregnancy:** Managing glucose resistance is essential for lowering the chance of developing type 2 diabetes in the future. Maintaining a healthy weight and remaining physically active can be beneficial lifestyle improvements.

Anemia in Pregnancy

- **Risk Factors:** Anemia is caused by a lack of red blood cells or hemoglobin. Inadequate iron intake, numerous pregnancies, and a history of anemia are all risk factors for anemia during pregnancy.
- **Symptoms:** Fatigue, weakness, pale complexion, and shortness of breath are common symptoms. In severe cases, anemia can cause dizziness, fast heartbeat, and difficulty focusing.
- **Chronic vs. Acute symptoms:** Chronic anemia develops slowly and has milder symptoms. Acute anemia, on the other hand, can strike unexpectedly and cause more severe symptoms.

- **Treatment:** Treatment mainly consists of iron supplements and dietary modifications. The proper treatment will be determined by your healthcare provider based on the degree of your anemia.
- **Prevention:** Pregnant women are generally advised to adopt an iron-rich diet, take prenatal vitamins, and follow their healthcare provider's iron supplementation guidelines to prevent anemia.

Worsening Heartburn

- **Cause:** Heartburn is prevalent during pregnancy as a result of hormonal changes and the developing uterus placing pressure on the stomach, resulting in acid reflux.
- **Symptoms:** Heartburn symptoms include a burning sensation in the chest, esophagus, or stomach, as well as reflux of stomach acid.
- **Management:** Eating smaller, more frequent meals, avoiding spicy and acidic foods, elevating your upper body while sleeping, and considering antacids that are safe to use during pregnancy are all recommended ways to control heartburn during pregnancy. Before taking any drugs, check with your healthcare provider.
- **Duration:** Heartburn can last or worsen during pregnancy, so it is important to treat it as needed for comfort.

Regular prenatal checkups during the second trimester are essential for monitoring your health and addressing any medical issues, ensuring a healthy pregnancy for you and your baby. As you progress into the third trimester, the focus shifts to preparing for the baby's birth, with notable physical changes and anticipation for labor and delivery. If you have any concerns or odd symptoms while pregnant, always consult your healthcare professional.

Third Trimester Overview

If I had my life to live over, instead of wishing away nine months of pregnancy, I'd have cherished every moment and realized that the wonderment growing inside me was the only chance in life to assist God in a miracle.

— Erma Bombeck

The third trimester of pregnancy is a remarkable phase marked by significant changes and challenges for expectant mothers. As the journey toward childbirth nears its culmination, a host of physical changes and skin-related issues emerge. During this time, your body adapts in unique ways to accommodate the growing life within, bringing both wonders and challenges that need attention and care.

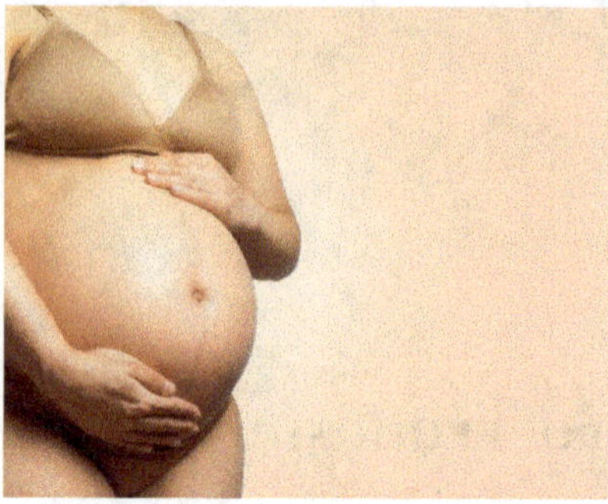

Linea nigra

Skin Concerns

Stretch marks: Stretch marks are common during pregnancy due to the stretching of the skin. They often appear as reddish or purplish streaks and can disappear with time. You can help avoid them by frequently moisturizing your skin using stretch mark prevention creams or oils.

Vein distension: As your uterus expands, it can exert pressure on blood vessels, causing vein distension, particularly in the legs. To ease discomfort, raise your legs whenever possible and wear support stockings if your healthcare professional recommends them.

Why is the skin on the belly darker in late pregnancy? This happens due to hormonal changes; the skin on the belly may grow darker in late pregnancy. This condition is known as chloasma or melasma. It's a temporary condition that normally fades after childbirth.

Why is there a dark line running down the middle of my baby bump? The dark line that runs down the center of your baby bump is known as "linea nigra". It is a result of increased pigmentation caused by hormonal changes and usually disappears postpartum.

Protruding Belly Buttons

During pregnancy, a protruding belly button is generally caused by the enlarging uterus pushing against the abdominal wall. This is not usually permanent and should return to normal following childbirth.

Gastrointestinal Concerns

- **Constipation:** Hormonal changes and pressure from the developing uterus might cause your digestive system to slow down, resulting in constipation. Increase your fiber intake, drink plenty of water, and engage in regular physical activity to combat this. Before using nonprescription laxatives, it is advisable to seek guidance from your healthcare professional.
- **Hemorrhoids:** Hemorrhoids refer to enlarged blood vessels in the rectal region. Pain, itching, and bleeding are all possible symptoms. To relieve symptoms, use over-the-counter treatments, sitz baths, and practice proper hygiene. Severe cases may necessitate medical attention.
- **Anal fissures:** Anal fissures are tiny tears in the anus lining that can often be caused by passing hard stools. Symptoms include discomfort and the occurrence of bleeding when passing stool. Dietary adjustments,

topical medicines, and, in severe cases, surgery are all possible treatments.

- **Umbilical hernia:** An umbilical hernia is a condition in which a part of the intestine protrudes through a weakness in the abdominal wall near the navel. Symptoms may include a bulge or soreness. In some cases, these hernias may be cured on their own after pregnancy, but surgery may be necessary in severe cases.

General Skin Care During Pregnancy

- **Hydration:** Maintain skin hydration by consuming an ample amount of water.
- **Sun protection:** Apply sunscreen to your skin to protect it from the sun, as it becomes more sensitive during pregnancy. Dermatologists recommend sunscreen of SPF at least 30, which is expected to block about 97% of the sun's UVB rays.
- **Moisturize:** To prevent dryness and itching, use a gentle, pregnancy-safe moisturizer.
- **Gentle cleansing:** To avoid skin irritations, use gentle, fragrance-free cleansers.
- **Avoid harsh chemicals:** When purchasing skincare products, avoid ones that include harsh chemicals or ingredients that may be unsafe during pregnancy.

Chapter 11

Pregnancy Month 7 (Weeks 27–30)

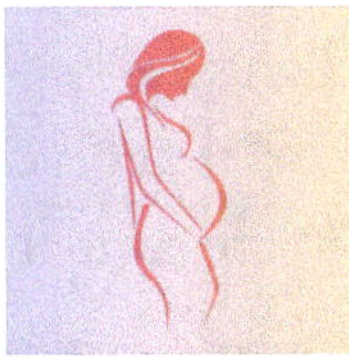

During the seventh month of pregnancy (weeks 27–30), your baby continues to grow rapidly, making a well-balanced diet even more important. To help your baby's bone development, choose calcium and vitamin D-rich foods such as dairy products and fortified cereals. In order to prevent anemia and encourage healthy blood circulation, increase intake of iron-rich foods such as lean meats and leafy greens. Finally, eat plenty of fiber from fruits, vegetables, and whole grains to avoid constipation, which is a common issue during this trimester.

11.1: Your Baby's Developmental Milestones in the Seventh Month

Your baby meets critical growth milestones in the seventh month of pregnancy. During this time, the baby's brain and sensory systems continue to develop, while its physical growth and appearance alter dramatically, setting the foundation for a healthy birth.

Brain and Nervous System Development

- The baby's brain undergoes rapid growth.
- The nervous system develops to the point where it can control some body functions.
- Hearing is fully developed and the baby can respond to sound, pain, and light.
- By weeks 29–30, the fetal brain can control body temperature and regulate regular breathing.

Sensory and Visual Development

- During this month, your baby's eyelids can open and close.
- The fetus can open its eyes, blink, and has eyelashes by week 27.
- The eyes might open wide by the end of the seventh month.
- Toenails begin to form.

Physical Growth and Weight Gain

- The fetus continues to grow and develop existing organs and systems during this month.
- The formation of subcutaneous fat for body insulation and general growth begins.
- The fetus is approximately 14 to 15 inches long and weighs between two and three pounds by the end of the seventh month.

Lung Development

- During weeks 27–30, the lungs continue to grow and develop in preparation for breathing after delivery.
- By weeks 29–30, the fetal brain can control normal breathing.

Fetal Mobility and Reflexes

- The baby often shifts positions, showing enhanced mobility.
- By weeks 29–30, the fetus can touch items weakly, demonstrating growing reflexes.

Amniotic Fluid and Survival Chances

- The amount of amniotic fluid that cushions the fetus begins to decrease as the baby grows larger.
- If your baby is born after week 27, he or she has a better chance of survival.

11.2 What to Expect This Month

The seventh month of pregnancy is a time of major physical and emotional changes for pregnant moms. Here's a rundown of what to expect during this stage.

Physical Changes

- **Pain:** Many women experience discomfort throughout the seventh month. This includes lower back pain due to the strain of an expanding belly.

Pressure on the sciatic nerve can result in hip and leg pain. Pelvic discomfort may also emerge as pelvic joints loosen in preparation for labor.

- **Breast changes:** Breasts may become more tender.
- **Skin sensitivity:** Hormones can cause skin sensitivity, dryness, flakiness, and possibly eczema. Stretch marks can appear on the belly, hips, and thighs. Varicose veins can form as a result of increased progesterone levels, but they normally disappear after birth.
- **Dizziness and fatigue:** Lightheadedness may be caused by pressure on blood vessels from the enlarging tummy. Fatigue can intensify as sleep becomes less restful in the third trimester.
- **Digestive and bladder issues:** High progesterone and iron levels can cause constipation and gas. Your baby's increased pressure may cause you to urinate more frequently.
- **Bleeding, spotting, and vaginal discharge:** While seeing light bleeding, spotting, or discharge during visits to the bathroom can be normal, it is wise to consult your healthcare provider. Gum irritation, edema, and bleeding may also occur during dental care.
- **Braxton-Hicks contractions:** Tightening of the abdomen, often referred to as Braxton-Hicks contractions, may occur. These are usually harmless practice contractions.

Emotional Adjustments

- **Fluctuating moods:** Hormones and physical changes can both cause mood swings.
- **Strengthening the parent-child bond:** Many pregnant parents feel a stronger connection with their unborn child during this month, but it's entirely okay if you don't; this connection often deepens post-delivery.
- **Anxiety:** Feeling anxious about what is to come is a normal response, but it is strongly recommended to seek professional help if you have feelings of extreme sadness or distress.

Medical Appointments

- **More frequent check-ups:** You will discover that you are probably going to the doctor more often during this period, usually every two weeks. These appointments involve monitoring your baby's growth, and activity, and assessing blood count and iron levels.
- **Tdap (Pertussis) vaccination:** It is crucial for pregnant women to receive the Tdap vaccine, preferably between 27 and 36 weeks of pregnancy. This vaccination provides a repository of immune cells that can be passed on to the baby, providing essential immunity against deadly diseases such as tetanus, diphtheria, and pertussis during the baby's first months of life (CDC, 2017).

- **Rh status assessment:** Rh-negative moms who are carrying Rh-positive babies may need Rh immune globulin injections (better known as Rhogam) to prevent immune system complications.
- **Breast changes:** Any breast changes, including the development of lumps, should be discussed with your healthcare provider.

How to Thrive at Seven Months Pregnant

- Prioritize sleep and try using a pregnancy pillow for extra support.
- Prenatal massages can help relieve discomfort.
- To stay active, continue with low-impact workouts.
- Maintain proper hydration and consume multiple small, fiber-rich meals to deal with gastric issues.
- Promptly discuss any physical or emotional issues with your healthcare provider.
- Begin researching hospitals and write down your birth plan in readiness for labor.

11.3: Gender—To Reveal or Not to Reveal?

The decision on whether to have a gender reveal party or not is a personal one, and it is important to consider various factors before making a decision. Here are some points to assist you in deciding whether or not to reveal your baby's gender at a party.

Pros of Having a Gender Reveal Party

- **Celebration:** Gender reveal parties allow pregnant parents to celebrate the imminent addition to their family with friends and relatives.
- **Excitement:** It can add an extra layer of excitement and anticipation to the prenatal process.
- **Involvement:** Gender reveal parties often include loved ones, allowing them to share in the joy and excitement of the occasion.
- **Memorable:** It can be a memorable event for everyone present to cherish, especially if it includes creative and fun reveal methods.
- **Gifts:** Guests enjoy bringing gifts for the baby, which might be useful for new parents.

Cons of Having a Gender Reveal Party

- **Pressure:** Some people may feel compelled to conform to social standards and throw a gender reveal party, even if they would prefer not to.
- **Gender stereotypes:** Gender reveal events might perpetuate traditional gender stereotypes because they often include gender-related themes and colors.
- **Overshadowing:** The gender reveal party may overshadow the more significant event of childbirth.
- **Diminishes excitement of the unknown:** Some expectant parents desire to be surprised by the gender of their child.
- **Environmental impact:** Some elaborate gender reveal ideas involve potentially dangerous practices,

such as fireworks or balloon releases, which can have a negative impact on the environment.

Alternative Options

If you choose not to have a gender reveal party or want to have a different approach, consider the following alternatives:

- **Private reveal:** You can find out the gender privately and inform only close family or friends.
- **Gender-neutral theme:** If you still want to celebrate, try a gender-neutral theme that emphasizes the joy of pregnancy rather than gender norms.
- **Wait until birth:** Some parents want to keep the baby's gender a secret until delivery, savoring the surprise.
- **Virtual reveal:** In today's digital age, the gender reveal moment can be shared with loved ones through a virtual event or video call.

Ultimately, your decision to have a gender reveal party should be based on your values and preferences, ensuring a memorable pregnancy experience. Remember, there are no right or wrong choices; what matters most is your comfort and happiness during this special time. Moving into the eighth month, get ready for the next chapter in your journey toward motherhood, drawing closer to the momentous day of childbirth after experiencing physical and emotional changes throughout the seventh month.

Chapter 12

Pregnancy Month 8 (Weeks 31–34)

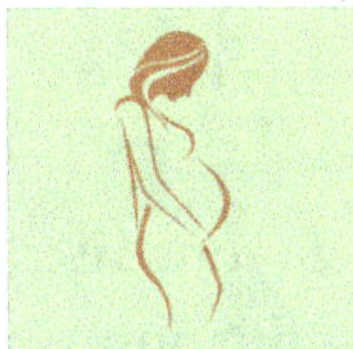

You are now in the final stretch, and you can expect a surge in the baby's activity, while also experiencing increased pressure and discomfort as the baby continues to grow. Fetal development will focus on improving organ functions, particularly the lungs, in preparation for the grand debut.

12.1: Your Baby's Developmental Milestones in the Eighth Month

The developmental milestones for the fetus will be discussed next.

Physical Development

Size and weight: By the eighth month, your baby is about 18 inches long and weighs around 5 pounds (American Pregnancy Association, n.d.-b). This signifies substantial growth in size and weight.

Skin and appearance:

- The fetus's skin is no longer transparent, indicating increased skin thickness.
- More fat accumulates under the skin, giving the fetus the appearance of a newborn baby.
- The lanugo hairs on the face start disappearing.

Muscle tone: Fetal muscle tone rises, indicating the development of strength and coordination.

Sensory and Brain Development

Vision: At this time, the baby can see. The pupils of the eyes react to light, showing that visual responsiveness is developing.

Brain development: Rapid development of the brain continues, signifying cognitive growth and maturation.

Stimulation response: The fetus can process more information and stimuli and you may detect more distinct patterns in its wakefulness and when it's asleep. This is an indication of a growing ability to respond to external stimuli.

Lungs: While most internal organs and systems are fully matured, the lungs still require time to develop. However, they continue to grow and produce surfactant, which aids in keeping the lungs open if the fetus is delivered prematurely (*Embryonic & fetal development*, 2015).

Ears: The ears retain their shape when moved, indicating the continued development of the auditory system.

Motor Skills

Movement: The baby's movements become more prominent as they begin to kick more, displaying developing motor skills.

Physiological Changes

Hiccups: During this period of development, the fetus may begin to have hiccups, which is a normal physiological occurrence.

12.2: What to Expect This Month

At eight months pregnant, here's what you can expect.

Emotional Changes

It is normal to feel a variety of feelings during this month, including excitement, anxiety, and anticipation about becoming a parent. It is important to acknowledge and address these feelings through caring for yourself.

Self-Care

Making time for yourself is essential. Virtual hangouts with friends, having a manicure and pedicure, meditation, and prenatal yoga can all help you relax and unwind. This author has a published book of targeted mindful meditations specifically curated for the self-care of expectant moms and new moms. Be sure to visit the Author Page for this book on Amazon and check out this amazing meditation resource and other essential publications to enhance your pregnancy journey.

Physical Changes

- **Shortness of breath:** As your uterus grows, it might press against your lungs, resulting in shortness of breath. Maintaining proper posture can make it easier to breathe.
- **Increased urination:** Pressure on your bladder from the baby shifting lower can cause more frequent trips to the bathroom.
- **Pelvic pressure:** As the baby descends lower into your pelvis in preparation for birth, you may feel pressure in your pelvic area.
- **Skin stretching:** Stretch marks may occur as your tummy grows larger. The use of lotions and creams on a regular basis can help avoid them.
- **Braxton-Hicks contractions:** As your due date approaches, you may experience more of these practice contractions.
- **Varicose veins:** Increased blood circulation, particularly in the legs, can result in varicose veins. Compression hosiery, such as socks or stockings, could be beneficial.
- **Hemorrhoids:** These are enlargements of the veins in the lower abdomen. They can be avoided by eating fiber-rich foods and staying hydrated.
- **Dizziness:** This can be reduced by standing up slowly and keeping consistent blood sugar levels through regular meals.
- **Fatigue:** This is the result of carrying extra weight and difficulty finding a comfortable sleeping posture.

Pregnancy pillows have been shown to help with sleep.

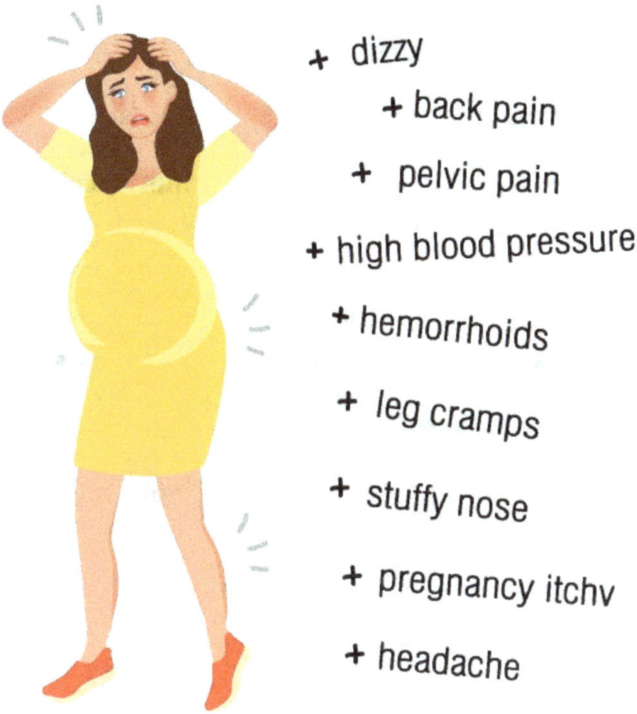

Weight Gain

On average, you should gain about a pound a week during the eighth month of pregnancy (Crider, 2021). However, this varies from person to person, so check with your doctor if you have concerns.

Baby's Position

As you approach delivery, your baby will settle into your pelvis, which may ease pregnancy heartburn. By the end of the month, your baby will most likely be head down. If not, your doctor may recommend strategies to urge the baby to turn.

Baby's Movements

You may feel less frequent but stronger movements from your baby because they have less room to stretch. Consult your doctor if you have any concerns regarding the nature or frequency of your baby's motions. They may recommend kick counts or diagnostic examinations.

When to See a Doctor

As your due date approaches, you'll see your midwife or OB-GYN more often. They will keep an eye on your and the baby's health. Contact your doctor right away if you experience

- your water breaking
- vaginal bleeding or infection symptoms
- frequent contractions or early signs of labor
- extreme vomiting or diarrhea
- preeclampsia symptoms like headaches, visual issues, and swelling in the hands and face.

Remember that every pregnancy has its own experience, so don't hesitate to reach out to your healthcare provider if you have any concerns or questions.

12.3: Birthing Plans

Expectant mothers can choose from a variety of birth plans and possibilities, each tailored to their specific preferences and needs. Here are some examples of common birthing plans:

- **Traditional hospital birth:** Many women want to have their babies in a hospital setting. Hospitals have readily available medical facilities, qualified staff, and emergency services. Traditional hospital birth is an excellent birthing option for pregnant women who want access to pain relief solutions such as epidurals.
- **Birthing centers in hospitals:** Some hospitals have birthing centers in-house. These facilities strive to provide a more homelike, comfortable setting for childbirth while still providing fast access to medical assistance if necessary.
- **Home birth:** Opting for a home birth alongside a skilled midwife offers a personalized and tranquil delivery experience. However, it is crucial to have a contingency plan ready for any potential complications.
- **Independent birthing centers:** These facilities cater to pregnancies with low risks, offering a compromise between home deliveries and hospital births. Staffed by midwives, they create a cozy atmosphere while remaining equipped to handle emergency situations.
- **Water birth:** Some women, whether in a birthing center or even at home, prefer to have a water birth.

During labor, the buoyancy of the water can provide pain relief and relaxation.

- **Unmedicated birth:** Many women choose an unmedicated birth, relying on breathing methods, movement, and the assistance of a doula or partner. This method avoids the use of pain medication and medical procedures.
- **Planned C-section:** This may be recommended by the healthcare provider or selected by the pregnant patient in certain instances. This could be for medical reasons, previous C-sections, or personal preference.
- **Doula-assisted birth:** Doulas are trained professionals who support mothers emotionally and physically during labor and childbirth. They can be invaluable members of the birthing team, offering guidance and comfort.
- **Hypnobirthing:** This method uses self-hypnosis and relaxation techniques to alleviate pain and promote a calm birthing experience.
- **Epidural or spinal block:** To reduce pain during delivery, some women choose pain treatment options like epidurals or spinal blocks. These are usually administered in a hospital setting.
- **Natural birth in a hospital:** Some hospitals offer "low-intervention" or "natural birth" programs. These aim to minimize medical interventions while still being in a hospital setting for safety.
- **Family-centered birth:** This approach encourages partners and family members to participate in the birthing process, making it a more inclusive experience.

When deciding on a birthing plan, it is essential to discuss your options with your healthcare provider, midwife, or doula. Based on your medical history, preferences, and the level of risk connected with your pregnancy, they can help you make informed decisions. Keep in mind that as birth can be unpredictable, flexibility is key. Therefore, your plans may need to adapt to changing conditions for the health and safety of both you and your baby.

12.4: Birthing Classes—What Are They?

Birthing classes are educational programs that help expectant parents prepare for childbirth and the postpartum period. These programs seek to equip expectant women and couples with information, practical skills, and emotional support to help them feel more confident and prepared for the birthing experience. Birthing classes vary in content and format, but they commonly address the following topics.

Labor and delivery education: Birthing classes often include information about the phases of labor, what to expect during each stage, and how labor proceeds. This can include discussions about labor signs, contraction timing, and when to go to the hospital or birthing center.

Pain management techniques: Many birthing classes teach various pain management strategies, both medicated and unmedicated. This may include relaxation exercises, breathing methods, visualization, and information on pain relief choices like epidurals.

Comfort measures: Birthing programs often focus on comfort measures that a partner or other members of the pregnant mom's support team can offer during labor, such as massage, positioning, and emotional support.

Medical interventions: Information about common medical interventions used during childbirth, such as inductions, C-sections, and fetal monitoring, may be discussed in birthing classes. This assists parents in understanding their options and making informed decisions.

Breastfeeding and postpartum care: Some birthing classes widen their scope to include the basics of breastfeeding and postpartum care for both the mother and baby.

Coping with unexpected outcomes: Some birthing classes include possible issues or unanticipated outcomes, as well as how to deal with them emotionally and medically.

Are Birthing Classes Necessary?

The necessity for birthing classes varies from person to person and pregnancy to pregnancy. Consider the following points.

First-time parents: Birthing lessons can be especially helpful for first-time parents who have no prior childbirth experience. They provide useful knowledge and help to ease anxiety about the unknown.

Knowledge and preparation: If you want a proper understanding of the birthing process, pain management options, and what to expect during labor and delivery, birthing classes can be very useful.

Partner involvement: For partners or support persons, birthing classes are an opportunity to learn how to actively participate in the birthing process, offering valuable support to the laboring person.

Specific circumstances: If you have particular concerns or are planning on having an unconventional birth, such as a home birth or water birth, specialized birthing classes can give you personalized guidance.

Community and networking: Birthing classes can offer a sense of community and an opportunity to interact with other pregnant women. This network of support can be quite beneficial during pregnancy and postpartum.

Personal comfort: Some people like to be as knowledgeable as possible about the delivery process and birthing classes help them feel more prepared and confident.

Nevertheless, birthing classes are not a must, and some people choose not to attend them. They choose to rely on other sources of information, like books, online resources, or discussions with their healthcare provider. In the end, whether or not you choose to take birthing classes is a personal decision, based on your individual needs, preferences, and circumstances. If you have specific questions or concerns regarding childbirth, go ahead and discuss them with your healthcare provider, who can help you make an informed decision.

12.5: Lamaze Breathing Techniques

Lamaze breathing techniques are a set of relaxation and breathing exercises used during labor and childbirth to assist in managing pain, reducing stress, and increasing control and focus. These practices are part of the Lamaze method, a prominent childbirth education program that teaches expecting mothers how to be more active and confident throughout labor and delivery (Lothian, 2011). Lamaze breathing techniques are often taught in childbirth programs, but they can also be performed on their own. Here are a few examples of common Lamaze breathing techniques:

Slow, deep breathing: This technique entails inhaling slowly through the nose and expelling slowly through the mouth. It aids in increasing oxygen flow to the body and relieving tension.

Patterned breathing: For moderate contractions, Lamaze recommends using particular rhythmic breathing patterns. Typical patterns include

- **Cleansing breath:** Take a deep cleansing breath before each contraction to alleviate tension.
- **Slow-paced breathing:** Inhale for four counts and exhale for six counts. This aids in maintaining focus and relaxation.
- **Pant-pant-blow:** Two quick, shallow breaths, followed by a prolonged expiration on the third count. This can aid with pain management during contractions (American Pregnancy Association, n.d.-d).

Breathing awareness: During labor, Lamaze emphasizes the significance of remaining connected to your breath and being aware of your body's sensations. Breathing awareness allows you to stay in the present moment and better manage discomfort.

Visualization: Along with breathing, Lamaze recommends adopting positive images and visualization techniques. Visualize a serene, pleasant environment or your baby descending through the delivery canal. Visualization might assist you in shifting your focus away from pain and anxiety (Frothingham, 2018).

Relaxation techniques: In addition to breathing, Lamaze supports a variety of relaxation techniques, including progressive muscular relaxation, massage, and posture modifications, in addition to breathing. These approaches can help you relax and feel more at ease.

Partner support: Lamaze encourages the birthing partner to play an active role in assisting the laboring person in practicing breathing methods. Partners can offer physical support and encouragement and remind the laboring person to breathe deeply and rhythmically.

Labor coping tactics: Lamaze offers coping tactics other than breathing, such as movement, changing positions, and finding comfort measures that work for you.

However, it is worth mentioning that while Lamaze breathing techniques can be beneficial, not all expectant mothers find them effective or necessary. Every labor experience is unique and what works well for one person may not work for another. The goal is to explore different coping strategies, attend birthing classes to learn and practice these techniques and remain adaptable during labor to your changing needs and comfort.

12.6: Alexander Birthing Techniques for Muscular Tension Release Through Sitting, Standing, and Movement

Alexander technique is a method developed by F. Matthias Alexander (1869–1955) to improve posture, movement, and overall well-being by dealing with muscular tension and improper use of the body. Despite it not being specifically a birthing technique, pregnant women can benefit from learning and practicing the Alexander Technique to relieve muscular tension and promote a more comfortable pregnancy and childbirth experience (Banoofatemeh et al., 2017). Here are some methods to apply the Alexander Technique concepts to sitting, standing, and movement during pregnancy.

Sitting

- **Use a chair with good support:** Select a chair with adequate back support and sit with your feet flat on the floor.
- **Avoid slouching:** Pay attention to your seating posture. Allow your spine to stretch and instead of rounding your back, sit on your sitting bones.
- **Practice mindful sitting:** Use the Alexander Technique principles to become aware of needless muscular tension. While seated, relax any tightness in your neck, shoulders, and back.

Standing

- **Weight distribution:** Distribute your body weight evenly between both feet. Avoid unnecessarily locking your knees or arching your lower back.
- **Stretch your spine:** Visualize your spine stretching from the crown of your head to your tailbone. This will assist you in maintaining a more upright and relaxed posture.
- **Release tension:** Pay attention to any areas of tightness, like the neck, shoulders, or lower back, and strive to let go of muscular tension that you do not need.
- **Mindful walking:** When walking during pregnancy, pay attention to your gait and balance. Avoid excessive swaying or striding.
- **Steady steps:** Instead of jerky or rapid movements, aim for smooth, coordinated steps that incorporate your entire body.
- **Breathe deeply:** Deep, diaphragmatic breathing should be incorporated into your movements. This can assist in alleviating stress and promoting relaxation.

Incorporating the Alexander Technique into your daily routine can improve body awareness, posture, and movement during pregnancy and labor.

12.7: Water Birthing—What Is It?

Water birthing is a way of giving birth in a birthing pool or tub filled with warm water. Expectant moms may choose this strategy if they believe that the buoyancy and warmth of the water will provide a more soothing and comfortable delivery experience. Here are several important aspects of water birth:

The Water Birthing Process

- Water childbirth involves a laboring woman entering a birthing pool or tub at various phases of labor, including the early stages of contractions and, in some cases, the actual delivery.
- Warm water is thought to calm the mother and relieve pain and strain on the body.
- Typically, the baby is born underwater and gently brought to the surface by the midwife or healthcare practitioner.

Celebrities Who Have Used Water Birthing

Celebrities such as supermodel Gisele Bündchen, actress Jacqueline Jossa, and Thandie Newton have all used water birthing during their deliveries. Gisele Bündchen gave birth to her son Benjamin at home in a water birth and underlined the lack of discomfort during the labor. She spoke about her desire for a drug-free and peaceful birth experience, having achieved this through prenatal yoga and meditation.

Jacqueline Jossa was enthusiastic about water childbirth, calling it "amazing." She couldn't bear the thought of giving birth on a bed and underlined the advantages of gravity when immersed in water. Thandie Newton had a positive experience with water childbirth as well, recognizing the difficult yet gratifying nature of the procedure. She expressed a wish to go through the process again, emphasizing the tremendous connection and vigor she felt throughout childbirth (Atkin, n.d.).

Advantages

- **Pain relief:** Many women find that immersing themselves in warm water helps to relieve pain and discomfort during delivery.
- **Relaxation:** Water's soothing impact helps induce relaxation, which can contribute to a more positive childbirth experience.
- **Buoyancy:** Being buoyant in water might help the mother move around and find comfortable postures during labor.
- **Reduction in interventions:** Some proponents argue that water delivery can reduce the requirement for medical interventions such as epidurals or episiotomies.

Risks

- **Infection:** If the water is not kept at the right temperature or the birthing pool is not properly cleaned, there is a danger of infection (Santilli, 2023).
- **Fetal distress:** Monitoring the baby's heart rate underwater can be difficult and fetal discomfort may not be immediately apparent.
- **Complications:** In rare cases, complications such as umbilical cord issues or meconium (baby's first stool) in the water can cause problems.

- **Maternal overheating:** Prolonged exposure to very hot water can result in maternal overheating, which can be harmful.

Current Evidence-Based Research

The research evidence on water birthing is conflicting (Harper, 2014).

Due to insufficient data on the safety and efficacy of water delivery, the American College of Obstetricians and Gynecologists (ACOG) and the American Academy of Pediatrics (AAP) have released guidelines cautioning against giving birth underwater.

Ultimately, the choice of birthing method, including water delivery, should be based on individual preferences, medical history, and consultation with a healthcare expert who can advise on what is safest and most appropriate for the mother and baby.

12.8: Hypnobirthing

Hypnobirthing is a method of preparing for childbirth that incorporates various relaxation and mindfulness practices to lessen fear, pain, and anxiety during labor and delivery. This practice emphasizes the mind-body link and tries to assist pregnant moms in having a more peaceful and happy birth experience. Some of the most important aspects that encompass hypnobirthing are

- **Positive affirmations:** These are statements or phrases that moms repeat to themselves in order to cultivate a positive attitude about birthing. They can assist in the replacement of negative thoughts with powerful and reassuring ones.

- **Guided meditation:** These sessions are often used to induce a state of deep relaxation. They can assist moms in remaining focused and calm during labor.
- **Visualization:** Visualization techniques assist mothers in visualizing a painless and easy birth. This can help in alleviating anxiety and stress.
- **Deep breathing:** Deep breathing exercises aid in the management of pain and stress during labor. Controlled and rhythmic breathing can help promote relaxation and reduce discomfort.

The effectiveness of hypnobirthing for pain management during labor remains inconclusive. While a research study has suggested the positive effects of hypnobirthing on fear, pain, satisfaction, and birth outcomes, overall evidence remains insufficient to firmly establish it as a reliable technique (Buran & Aksu, 2022). Therefore, caution is advised and decisions should be made in conjunction with healthcare experts taking into account individual preferences and needs.

12.9: The Bradley Method of Natural Childbirth

This method, developed by Dr. Robert Bradley, stresses that natural childbirth is possible without the use of medication and favors the idea that a woman can give birth with the help of her partner. Here's a brief overview of the method and some scientific views.

- **Natural childbirth focus:** The Bradley method emphasizes natural childbirth, focusing on relaxation, deep breathing, and natural pain management strategies above medical treatments such as epidurals or medications.
- **Partner involvement:** A key aspect of this technique is the active participation of the birthing woman's husband, partner, or coach. Partners are taught how to provide physical and emotional support during labor and delivery.
- **Education and preparation:** Women and their partners are advised to undergo comprehensive childbirth education sessions to better understand the labor and delivery process. This involves learning about anatomy, labor stages, and pain management techniques.

Scientific Views

The Bradley method of birthing lacks strong scientific evidence to conclusively support its efficacy over other childbirth preparation strategies (Gurevich, 2021). While some people may find it useful, the scientific community generally believes that more rigorous research is needed to determine its genuine value in improving maternal and neonatal outcomes.

Choosing how to give birth is a personal decision that should prioritize the health of both mom and baby. Discuss options with your prenatal care team and choose a hospital that meets your needs. As you move from the eighth to the ninth month, get ready for the final stretch—preparations, signs of labor, and the thrilling moments leading up to childbirth!

Chapter 13

Pregnancy Month 9 and Up (Weeks 35–40)

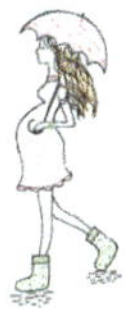

Welcome to the ninth and final month of pregnancy, an exciting and crucial time as you prepare for your baby's arrival! During this final stretch, your baby is rapidly gaining weight and preparing for life outside the womb. It is essential to focus on a well-balanced diet that delivers the required nutrients for both your and your baby's health.

13.1: "Ready to Pop"—Am I Going to Be Pregnant Forever?

This phrase often crosses the minds of expectant mothers as they enter the ninth month of pregnancy. It is natural to feel impatient and uncomfortable during this time but rest assured, you won't be pregnant forever! These last few weeks of pregnancy, however difficult, are worthwhile for various reasons.

- **Development of vital organs:** The final weeks of pregnancy are crucial for the development of your baby's organs, notably the lungs and brain. The baby is rapidly growing and fine-tuning vital systems as it prepares for life outside the womb. This time period ensures that your baby is born with the highest possible health and well-being.

- **Weight gain and nutritional reserve:** Your baby is gaining weight quickly in these final weeks. This extra weight is necessary for maintaining body temperature and conserving nutrients during the first few days after birth, when breastfeeding may not be fully established. It acts as a nutritional reserve, allowing your baby to thrive in the early stages of life.
- **Formation of bond:** The latter weeks of pregnancy provide you with unique opportunities to bond with your unborn child. You can talk to your baby, feel their movements, and form a strong bond with them. These are tremendously rewarding moments that will serve as the foundation for your relationship as your child grows.
- **Maternal health:** While the final few weeks of pregnancy might be uncomfortable, your body is also preparing for childbirth. Your cervix is softening and dilating and your uterine muscles are practicing contractions. These physiological changes are necessary for a smoother labor and delivery process.
- **Psychological preparation:** The final few weeks of pregnancy provide you with the opportunity to mentally and emotionally prepare for motherhood. You may use this time to take childbirth and parenting classes, read books, and connect with other expectant parents. This preparation can serve to

enhance your confidence and readiness to welcome your baby into the world.

So, while it's natural to want to meet your baby and be relieved of the physical discomforts of late pregnancy, try to focus on these important reasons why the last few weeks are worth the wait. It's a fantastic and transformational time in your life and before you know it, you'll be holding your precious newborn infant in your arms, making all the difficulties of the final stretch of your pregnancy seem worthwhile. Remember that your healthcare provider is there to help you through this journey and if you have any concerns or questions regarding the final weeks of pregnancy, don't hesitate to contact them for advice and reassurance.

13.2: Your Baby's Developmental Milestones This Month

In the ninth month of pregnancy, your baby is undergoing remarkable changes in preparation for life outside the womb. This month is marked by key developmental milestones, ranging from lung maturation to physical changes, positioning for birth, and the thrilling transition to full-term pregnancy, all of which contribute to your baby's readiness to embrace the world.

Lung Development and Maturation

- The lungs become mature in readiness for birth.
- Fetal lungs are almost always developed by weeks 37–38 after the last menstrual period (*Embryonic & fetal development*, 2015).

- This maturity is an indication of the baby being able to breathe independently upon birth.

Reflexes and Coordination

- Reflexes become more coordinated, making it possible for the baby to respond to sounds, blink, grasp, and turn their head (American Pregnancy Association, n.d.).
- These reflexes are essential for the baby's survival and adaptation to the outside world.

Fetal Positioning

- In preparation for birth, the baby moves into a head-down position near the birth canal.
- This positioning matters greatly for a more efficient delivery process.

Physical Changes

- Hair growth on the baby's head continues and lanugo (fine body hair) begins to fall off.
- Toenails grow all the way to the tip of the fetus's toes.
- More fat accumulates beneath the baby's skin, making them appear chubbier.

Sexual Development

- In male fetuses, testes begin to descend from the abdomen into the scrotum.

- The labia (vaginal lips) begin to cover the clitoris in female fetuses.

Final Growth Spurt

- In the latter weeks of pregnancy, the baby continues to grow rapidly, gaining roughly a half pound every week (Cleveland Clinic, 2023).
- Week 39 is considered a full-term pregnancy, and this is when the majority of babies are born.
- By the end of this month, the baby should weigh 7 to 9 pounds and be 18 to 20 inches long.
- This period shows that the baby is fully developed and ready to meet the world.

Onset of Labor

- At any point during this final month, you could go into labor, so it's essential to be prepared and vigilant for labor signs.
- As the baby descends toward the pelvis, you may feel increased pressure in your lower abdomen and pelvis.

13.3: What to Expect This Month

In the ninth month of pregnancy, here's what usually happens to mothers-to-be:

Physical Symptoms

- **Pain:** Your ever-expanding tummy may cause some discomfort, particularly in your back. Furthermore, your pelvic bones are loosening up in preparation for the big day, creating soreness.

- **Swelling:** Due to water retention, you may experience swelling in your legs, ankles, and feet. It's an excellent reason to sit back and unwind.
- **Frequent bathroom visits:** You can blame it on your growing uterus. You'll be using the bathroom more frequently and constipation may become an unwelcome guest.
- **Skin changes:** Be prepared for hyperpigmentation, blotchy areas, stretch marks, and maybe varicose veins.
- **Sleep struggles:** It can feel like an Olympic sport to find a comfortable sleeping posture. Your belly is to blame.

Breastfeeding Preparation

- **Breast leakage:** Your breasts may begin to produce colostrum, the first nourishment for your infant. It's normal, but if you notice anything out of the ordinary, consult your doctor.

Braxton-Hicks Contractions

You'll probably encounter more of these "practice contractions." Relax, they're just your body preparing for labor.

Emotional Changes

- **Nesting:** Suddenly, you'll experience a surge of energy and feel compelled to clean, organize, and

prepare your home for the new arrival. Nesting mode: activated!
- **Mood swings:** Due to lack of sleep, physical strain, and hormonal changes, your emotions may experience a rollercoaster ride.
- **Forgetfulness:** Don't be surprised if you're forgetful; it's commonly referred to as "pregnancy brain."

Doctor's Visits (Weekly)

- Doctor's visits and prenatal visits will now be scheduled on a weekly basis. Expect monitoring of blood pressure, weight, and fundal height.
- They'll monitor the fetal heartbeat and the position of the baby. If your baby is breech, your doctor may advise use of turning procedures or possibly have a C-section.
- Your cervix will be checked for dilation, and you may be tested for Group B Streptococcus, which is an infection that may necessitate antibiotics.

As we reach the end of the ninth month of pregnancy, which has been filled with both physical and emotional experiences, the focus is on the grand finale: labor and welcoming your baby. These milestones mark an incredible transformation, preparing both you and your baby for a successful birth.

Part Three

Labor and Preparing for Baby

There is a secret in our culture, and it is not that birth is painful. It's that women are strong.

— Laura Stavoe

Chapter 14

Time to Reap the Rewards

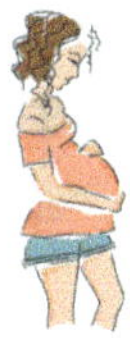

In Part III of the pregnancy journey, it is finally time to delve into the fruits of your labor and the preparations required for the arrival of your bundle of joy. It is time to reap the rewards of your hard work and dedication throughout this journey. From the trials you have succeeded in overcoming to the love and anticipation that fills your heart, this chapter marks a celebration of the beautiful moments and thoughtful preparations that come with the impending arrival of your precious baby.

14.1: Packing for the Hospital

Packing for the hospital is a memorable part of preparing for your baby's arrival. With various hospital policies, length of stay, and individual birth plans, it is important that you focus on what both you and your baby will require following the delivery, amidst all the advice and stories that you will be hearing from well-meaning individuals. This hospital bag packing list is intended to simplify the process and reduce your anxiety as you get ready for the upcoming labor and delivery.

General Guide for Packing

- **When to pack:** It is advisable to begin packing your hospital bags several weeks before your due date, just in case you go into labor early. This will also keep you from becoming overwhelmed and ensure you have all you need.
- **How to pack:** Pack your belongings in separate bags for easier access. To keep items orderly and visible, use clear plastic bags or packing cubes. Labeling your bags is also a good idea. Ensure that your bags are not too heavy, as you may have to transport your things on your own.

The Four Most Important Bags to Pack for the Hospital

Your personal/main bag: This bag will contain all the essentials for your comfort and delivery, such as

- Two easy slip-on gowns: Comfortable clothing that is easily worn and taken off.
- Two nightgowns: Comfy sleepwear.
- Two dressing gowns: Robes for additional comfort.
- Two pairs of socks: These will keep your feet nice and toasty.
- Disposable or comfortable underwear in dark colors.
- Take a dark-colored towel as it can get stained.
- Maternity-size sanitary pads that you will need for postpartum bleeding.

- A toothbrush and toothpaste are needed for your basic hygiene.
- Nursing bra in case you are planning to breastfeed.
- Breast pads to help with absorbing leaks.
- Nipple cream to provide nipple comfort.
- Cell phone and charger to help you stay connected.
- Other electronic gadgets for entertainment or communication, if you need them.
- Additional items to consider:
- Slippers or comfortable shoes.
- Post-delivery attire that is loose and comfy.
- Snacks or energy bars for a quick, nourishing snack.
- Books, magazines, or a tablet to help pass the time.
- Important documents such as your ID, insurance information, and birth plan.
- List of important contact numbers.

Labor mini-bag: This bag should contain items required for assistance during the labor process.

- Heating pads to help alleviate pain.
- Water bottle to keep you hydrated.
- Hair clips/scrunchies to ensure your hair is kept back from your face.
- Loose flannel gown/clothing is suitably comfortable attire for wearing during labor.
- Additional items to consider:
- Massage oil or lotion for a soothing effect.
- Stress-relief tools such as a stress ball, music, and aromatherapy.

- Birth plan, if you do not already have it in your main bag.
- Lip balm

Baby's bag: This will have all the items needed for your precious new arrival.

- Baby clothes for your newborn, onesies, baby sleepers, and outfits.
- Small, newborn-sized diapers.
- Baby wipes are needed for diaper changes.
- Diaper cream to help prevent diaper rash.
- Suction bulb to assist in clearing baby's nasal passages.
- Muslin cloths for swaddling your baby and for various cleaning purposes.
- Baby blanket to ensure your baby stays snug and comfortable.
- Baby accessories like caps, mittens, and vests can help keep your baby comfortable and cozy.
- Additional items to consider:
- Baby booties or socks.
- Pacifiers, if you are planning to use them.
- Baby book or journal for recording fond memories.

Spouse/partner bag: This needs to have the following essential items:

- Phone and charger for staying in touch with family and friends or other work requirements.

- Money (cash and credit card) to cover any unanticipated expenses.
- Food (snacks) to help maintain energy.
- Water and drinks are a vital requirement for staying hydrated.
- Change of clothing as your partner may need fresh clothes.
- A toothbrush and toothpaste are necessary hygiene items.
- Additional items to consider:
- Camera or video camera for capturing cherished moments.
- Book, magazine, or tablet to stay entertained and pass the time as the baby will definitely have their own schedule.
- Contact information for key people, including family and friends.

Should I Shave My Pubic Area for Labor?

Shaving your pubic area for labor is entirely up to you and there is no medical requirement. In fact, many healthcare providers advise against shaving the pubic area before labor. Shaving can lead to the risk of skin irritation and infection (Cummings, 2023).

Hospitals and healthcare professionals are well-prepared to manage labor and delivery without the need for shaving. If you are worried or have questions about grooming before labor, go right ahead and discuss them with your healthcare provider, who can provide proper guidance based on your specific condition and preferences. Ultimately, the decision should be yours, based on what makes you comfortable and what you believe is best for you.

14.2: Preparing An Older Child for New Baby's Arrival

Preparing an older child for the newest addition to the family requires a thoughtful approach, taking into account their age, temperament, and individual needs. Here are some steps and considerations to think about as you prepare your older child for their new sibling's arrival:

Communication and Explanation

- Share the news about the arrival of a new brother or sister with the older child in an age-appropriate and positive manner.
- Encourage the child to ask questions and give honest, straightforward responses.
- To help children understand the concept of becoming a sibling, read age-appropriate books or stories about it.

Involvement and Participation

- Encourage the child to help set up the baby's nursery or room and give them the chance to contribute ideas or decorations.
- Involve the child in helping to choose baby clothes, toys, or other items.
- Before the baby is delivered, encourage the child to talk to or sing to it while it is still in the womb. This will enable bonding between the two children.

Role-Playing and Pretend Play

- Perform short skits on feeding, diapering, and comforting using dolls or stuffed animals.
- You can teach kindness and care by pretending to be a doctor and having your little toddler examine the "baby" doll.

Emphasizing Their Importance

- Explain to your older child that they will soon be having a new role: that of being a "big brother" or "big sister."
- Make your older child feel important and smart by assigning small, age-appropriate tasks, such as laying out baby clothes or helping with the baby's bath.

Spending Quality Time

- Spending quality time with your older offspring helps to reassure them of your love and attention.
- Planning fun family activities together is a great way to strengthen the bond.

Managing Expectations

- Be explicit on the type of behavior you expect around the infant, such as being gentle and using indoor voices.
- Ensure your child fully understands and is well-prepared for the upcoming changes to the daily

routine that they will soon be facing. However, try to keep their personal routine as consistent as possible to provide stability, ensuring the older child gets adequate sleep and rest to deal with the adjustments.

Acknowledging Feelings

- **Open dialogue:** Encourage your child to speak up about their feelings. Ask them whether they are looking forward to the baby's arrival or have any fears or anxieties.
- **Validation:** Accept their emotions and let them know there is nothing wrong with how they are feeling.

Visiting the Hospital

- If possible, take your child with you when you go to the hospital and show them around to familiarize them with the setting and the location of the baby's birth.
- Arrange for the older child to meet their new sibling at the hospital, as this can be an exciting and bonding experience.

Gifts and Tokens of Affection

- Present the older sibling with a small gift or token from the baby upon their meeting.
- Consider establishing a reward system for good behavior or helpfulness during the transition period.

Patience and Reassurance

- Pay proper attention to the older child, reassuring them of your love, throughout the pregnancy and after the baby is born.
- Recognize the older child's positive behavior and cooperation, praising and thanking them for their effort.

Remember that every child is different, and how they may react to a new sibling can vary greatly. Be flexible and adjust your approach to your child's needs and responses. The aim is to cultivate a loving and positive relationship between your older child and the new baby.

14.3: Braxton-Hicks Versus Cramping Versus Real Labor Contractions

Expectant mothers need to have a clear understanding of the differences between Braxton-Hicks contractions, cramping, and true labor contractions as they get ready for childbirth. Here's a breakdown of each:

Braxton-Hicks Contractions

- **Characteristics:** These are commonly known as "practice contractions." They are usually irregular, sporadic, and lack a consistent pattern. They are milder than true labor contractions.
- **Timing:** You experience Braxton-Hicks contractions at any time during pregnancy, but they are commonly felt in the second and third trimesters.

- **Causes:** Dehydration, physical activity, or your baby's movements can all be possible causes.
- **Effect:** These contractions are normally not painful, just mildly uncomfortable. They do not cause cervical dilation and are not an indication of labor progression (Raines & Cooper, 2023).

Cramping

- **Characteristics:** The feeling of cramping in pregnancy is comparable to the experience you have with menstrual cramps or abdominal pain. It may feel like a dull aching or intermittent pain.
- **Timing:** Cramping can happen at any stage during pregnancy, with varying frequency and intensity.
- **Causes:** Cramping is triggered by a variety of factors, such as the stretching of the uterus, gas, constipation, or ligament pain.
- **Effect:** In most cases, cramping is temporary and not linked with labor contractions. It comes and goes and often gets better with rest, hydration, or shifting positions.

Real Labor Contractions

- **Characteristics:** True contractions are regular, become increasingly frequent, and get stronger and more painful over time. They follow a consistent pattern starting at the back and moving toward the front of the abdomen and have a duration of about 60 to 90 seconds (ACOG, 2020a).

- **Timing:** True labor contractions usually take place in the later stages of pregnancy, around the 37th week or later. They cause cervical dilation and effacement, which is the opening and thinning of the cervix.
- **Causes:** Hormonal changes and the body's preparation for delivery trigger true contractions.
- **Effect:** These are normally painful contractions and intensify as labor progresses. Instead of subsiding with rest, they continue and get closer together. Actual labor contractions are an indication that labor is underway, and it is time to head to the hospital or birthing center.

It is worth mentioning that everyone's experience with contractions and cramping is not necessarily the same. If you are not sure about what is causing your discomfort or contractions, you should contact your healthcare provider. They can properly guide you and help in determining whether you are having Braxton-Hicks contractions, cramping, or real labor contractions, and what to do next in light of your specific situation.

14.4: Third Trimester Vaginal Bleed—Is It a Cause for Concern?

A vaginal bleed during the third trimester of pregnancy is a concerning symptom that should not be ignored. While not all instances of bleeding are emergencies, it is crucial to take any bleeding seriously and seek medical attention promptly. Here are some possible causes of third-trimester vaginal bleeding, and why it should be evaluated by a healthcare provider

(Cleveland Clinic, 2021):

- **Placenta previa:** This happens when the placenta covers a portion or the entirety of the cervix. Bleeding in the third trimester, especially painless bleeding, can be a sign of placenta previa. This condition requires medical evaluation and may necessitate a cesarean section if it persists.
- **Placental abruption:** This involves a premature separation of the placenta from the wall of the uterus. Vaginal bleeding, abdominal pain, and contractions are all possible symptoms. Placental abruption is a medical emergency and should be treated immediately.
- **Cervical changes:** Some bleeding may be the result of cervix changes as it gets ready for labor, like cervical effacement or dilation. However, heavy or persistent bleeding should be properly examined by a healthcare provider.
- **Uterine rupture:** This is a rare but serious condition in which the uterine wall tears, potentially causing bleeding and exposing both the mother and the baby to risk. It often leads to emergency surgery.
- **Vaginal or cervical infections:** These infections can cause bleeding and should be treated promptly to prevent complications.
- **Trauma:** A pelvic injury or trauma might result in bleeding. It is essential to determine the cause and ensure everything is right with the baby.
- **Other causes:** Cervical polyps, sexually transmitted infections, and other medical disorders are among the

less prevalent causes of third-trimester bleeding. A healthcare provider can identify the cause through examination and testing.

If you have any vaginal bleeding during the third trimester of pregnancy, no matter how much or due to what circumstances, you should:

- **Seek immediate medical attention:** Get in touch with your healthcare provider or head toward the nearest hospital or birthing center. Do not delay, particularly if the bleeding is heavy, painful, or continuous.
- **Avoid certain activities:** Until the reason for the bleeding is determined, your healthcare provider may advise bed rest or limitations on all kinds of physical activity.
- **Stay hydrated:** Dehydration can worsen certain conditions linked to pregnancy, so it is important to drink water if advised by your healthcare provider.
- **Monitor fetal movement:** Monitor your baby's movements. Report any change in fetal activity to your doctor.

Remember that in cases of third-trimester bleeding, early detection, and prompt medical intervention can dramatically improve outcomes. It is always best to err on the side of caution and have a medical professional examine your situation.

14.5: Exercises to Promote Fetal Descent and Positioning

Promoting fetal descent and positioning is a crucial aspect in the achievement of a smooth and safe labor and delivery process. However, before you decide to undertake any exercise during pregnancy, consult with your healthcare provider, as individual circumstances may vary (ACOG, 2020). Here are several exercises and activities to help encourage fetal descent and positioning:

Pelvic Tilts (Cat-Cow Stretch)

- Assume a position on all fours, ensuring that your hands are positioned beneath your shoulders and your knees are aligned under your hips.
- Arch your back upward (cat pose) and then lower your back, buttocks protruding (cow pose).
- This exercise helps to ease back pain while encouraging the baby to move into a more favorable position.

Deep Squats

- Take up a standing position with your feet shoulder-width apart.
- Slowly squat down as far as possible, keeping your back straight and chest up.
- If necessary, hold on to a stable support.
- Deep squats can assist in opening up your pelvic area and encouraging your baby to drop in the pelvis.

Kegel Exercises

- Kegel exercises help to strengthen the pelvic floor muscles, helping the baby descend and get into optimal position.
- Kegels involve contracting your pelvic floor muscles, like when you are trying to stop the flow of urine, hold for a few seconds, and then let go.

Walking

- Walking helps prepare the cervix and increases the chances of spontaneous labor (Shojaei et al., 2021).
- Regular walking can help to gently lower the baby into the pelvis.
- Walking is helpful in alleviating the discomfort and pressure that often accompanies pregnancy.

Swimming

- Swimming and water aerobics are the kinds of low-impact sports that can help to reduce pressure on your pelvis while enhancing circulation and relaxation.

Prenatal Yoga

- Prenatal yoga can enhance flexibility and balance, promote relaxation, and encourage optimal fetal positioning (Yekefallah et al., 2021).

Pelvic Circles

- Maintain an erect posture while seated on either an exercise ball or a chair.
- Gently move your hips in a circular manner at a leisurely pace.
- This exercise aids in loosening the pelvic joints and promotes optimal positioning.

Child's Pose

- Kneel on the floor in a way that has your big toes touching and keep your knees apart.
- Sit back on your heels, slowly bend forward, and stretch your arms out in front of you.
- This pose can help reduce back and hip pain and encourage the baby to move into the pelvis.

Butterfly Stretch

- Sit in an upright position on the floor.
- Join the soles of your feet, keeping your knees bent outward.
- Now, as you pull your feet toward your body, you will feel your hips and inner thighs stretching.
- This stretch can assist in opening up your pelvis and getting the baby in a proper position.

Performing pelvic floor exercises with regularity can strengthen the muscles needed to support the baby's descent. It is important to note that your healthcare provider or a certified prenatal fitness instructor should always be consulted before starting any new workout routine during pregnancy. They can offer proper advice that aligns with your specific health situation.

You should also discuss any worries about the baby's posture with your healthcare practitioner, as they may suggest particular techniques or interventions to urge the baby to enter the optimal position for labor and delivery.

14.6: Types of Fetal Positioning

Fetal positioning has an important role during labor and childbirth. How easily labor progresses is hugely dependent on the position of the baby's head and body within the mother's pelvis. Here are various fetal positions (Chamberlain & Steer, 1999):

Occiput Anterior Position

- This is the ideal position in which the baby's head is down and facing the mother's back. The backside of the baby's head, referred to as the occiput, is positioned toward the front of the mother's pelvis.
- This is the most favorable position for smooth and efficient labor, as it enables the smallest part of the baby (the head) to enter the pelvis first.

Occiput Posterior Position

- The baby usually descends into the pelvis headfirst, with its face directed toward the mother's belly. The occiput is positioned toward her spine.

- Occiput posterior positions can prolong labor, making it more painful as the baby's head may have difficulty fitting through the pelvis.

Oblique Position

- This is when the baby's head is not fully engaged in the pelvis and is inclined at an angle.
- The oblique position may cause irregular contractions accompanied by lengthier and more difficult labor.

Transverse Position

- The baby lies in a sideways position across the mother's pelvis, with the head on one side and the feet on the other.
- Vaginal delivery is not appropriate with a transverse position and necessitates a cesarean section.

Breech Position (AKA Breech Presentation)

- In this position, the baby's buttocks or feet are positioned to emerge first instead of the head.
- Breech presentations can make delivery more difficult and riskier, and they often require a planned cesarean operation to protect the baby's health. However, under certain conditions, some healthcare professionals with breech delivery experience may attempt a vaginal birth.

It must be understood that fetal positioning is known to change during pregnancy and even in labor. While some positions are better than others for more comfortable labor and delivery, the baby's final position cannot always be predicted or influenced. During prenatal visits, healthcare providers monitor fetal positioning and may suggest techniques, exercises, or positions to urge the baby to shift into a more favorable presentation.

14.7: Vaginal Birth

Vaginal birth occurs when a baby leaves the mother's uterus, passing through the birth canal to be born by way of the vaginal opening. This process is also known as natural childbirth or vaginal delivery. It is the most common and safest method of childbirth and normally takes place in situations where both the mother and her baby are healthy and there are no complications involved that may require a cesarean section (C-section).

Advantages

Vaginal birth is a natural process, the way human bodies have evolved to give birth. It has several potential benefits for both the mother and her child.

- **Shorter recovery time:** In many cases, women who have had a vaginal birth recover more quickly than those who have been through a C-section. They also often report having experienced less pain and discomfort in the postpartum period.
- **Lower risk of complications:** Vaginal birth has a

lower risk of complications like infection, blood loss, and surgical issues that can emerge with a C-section.

- **Early bonding:** Mothers who have undergone a vaginal delivery may find it easier to initiate skin-to-skin contact and breastfeeding immediately after birth. This provides a better chance of bonding and breastfeeding success.
- **Lower cost:** Vaginal births are generally less expensive than C-sections, offering a more affordable choice for both individuals and healthcare systems.

Risks

- **Tearing or episiotomy:** A vaginal birth can result in the area between the vagina and anus, called the perineum, ripping. Sometimes to make the delivery process easier, healthcare providers may need to perform an episiotomy (a surgical cut) to widen the vaginal opening. Both of these situations can cause discomfort and require stitches.
- **Prolonged labor:** Some women have to endure labor for longer periods or may have stalled labor, resulting in exhaustion and the use of interventions like forceps or vacuum extraction.
- **Infection:** A vaginal birth is not without the risk of infection, especially if the amniotic sac has ruptured and there is an extended period of time between the water breaking and the actual birth.
- **Pelvic floor issues:** Vaginal birth may exert pressure and weaken the pelvic floor muscles. This can cause

future life disorders such as urinary incontinence or pelvic organ prolapse.
- **Fetal distress:** In some cases, the baby could be in distress during labor, prompting interventions like a vacuum extraction or emergency C-section.
- **Tissue damage:** There are rare cases of vaginal birth causing damage to the vaginal and perineal tissues, resulting in pain and possible future issues.

Remember that when deciding to have a vaginal birth, it is essential to have a proper consultation with a healthcare provider who will determine the specific conditions of the pregnancy, the mother's health, and the baby's position. Many factors, including existing complications, can affect the choice between vaginal birth and C-section. Healthcare providers work toward the safest and most appropriate delivery method for both the mother and the baby.

14.8: Labor Induction—Ways to Induce and Progress Labor

Planned Induction

This is the deliberate initiation of labor through medical interventions. It can be scheduled ahead of time for a variety of reasons, including post-term pregnancy, medical complications, or other concerns. It can also be used when labor is not proceeding as planned.

Pitocin (Synthetic Oxytocin)

- Pitocin is a synthetic version of oxytocin, a hormone that helps uterine contractions during labor.

- It can be administered through an IV drip to trigger contractions and progress labor.

Advantages: Pitocin can assist in inducing or increasing labor when required, potentially avoiding complications linked with prolonged labor.

Risks: Contractions can become overly strong or excessive, causing fetal distress and the need for a cesarean section. Overusing Pitocin can also enhance the risk of uterine hyper-stimulation (contractions that are excessive or prolonged).

Forceps Delivery

Forceps are medical instruments that look like tongs or salad servers and are employed during delivery to gently grasp the baby's head and guide the baby out of the birth canal.

Risks

- **Maternal discomfort:** Forceps can lead to some maternal discomfort or injury, in the form of bruising or tears.
- **Fetal injury:** There is a small risk of injury to the baby, such as bruises or marks on the baby's head, and more serious injuries in rare cases.
- **Trauma to the birth canal:** Forceps may generate vaginal or perineal cuts in the mother.
- **Increased risk of episiotomy:** An episiotomy may be needed to enable the use of forceps.

Pros

- **Facilitates vaginal delivery:** In situations involving concerns about prolonged labor or fetal distress, forceps can help guide the baby's head through the birth canal.
- **Diminishes the need for a cesarean section:** In some cases, forceps delivery can avoid the necessity for a more invasive cesarean section.
- **Reduces the second stage of labor:** Forceps can speed up the delivery procedure and lessen the amount of time the baby spends in the birth canal.

It is important to note that healthcare professionals will decide whether to use forceps during delivery based on the specific medical conditions. Forceps are often used when the benefits outweigh the dangers and when alternative delivery methods are proving to be unsafe for the mother or baby. Careful assessment and monitoring are required when undertaking forceps-assisted deliveries, ensuring that the well-being of both the mother and the newborn is not compromised.

14.9: Labor

Labor is a complicated process heralding the onset of childbirth. Here are some key points to help you properly understand labor.

Signs of True Labor

- **Contractions:** True labor contractions depict regularity, increased frequency, and intensity with time. They often feel like intense menstrual cramps that come and go at regular intervals, beginning in the lower back and spreading to the abdomen.

- **Bloody show:** A mucus-like discharge speckled with blood can be an indication of the cervix dilating. This is a key indicator of true labor.
- **Water breaking:** The amniotic sac ruptures, resulting in an outpouring or a slow leak of amniotic fluid. This can signal the beginning of labor or that it is already in progress.

Timing Labor Contractions

- Contractions can be timed using a stopwatch, a smartphone app, or a clock with a second hand.
- Start the timer when the contraction begins and stop when it ends.
- Note the duration (how much time each contraction takes) and the frequency (the time elapsing between the contractions).
- Timing contractions should start as soon as they become regular, which is usually when they occur about every 5 minutes and last around 60 seconds each.

Stages of Labor

- **Stage 1:** This is the longest and is separated into three phases: early labor (contractions become more regular and the cervix dilates), active labor (rapid dilation and stronger contractions), and transition (the cervix fully dilates, usually the most painful phase).

Cervical Effacement

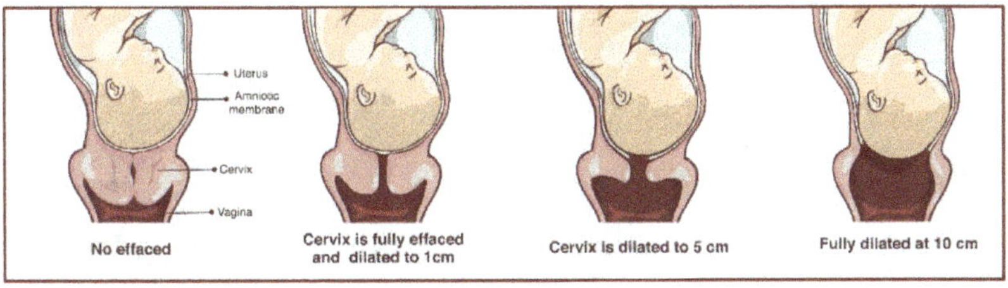

- **Stage 2:** This is the pushing phase, during which the baby passes through the birth canal.
- **Stage 3:** This is the phase of placenta delivery (afterbirth).

Breathing Techniques

- These techniques are often taught during delivery preparation classes.
- Practicing controlled and rhythmic breathing can help manage pain and anxiety during labor.
- Breathing techniques are often used during the active labor period when contractions are being felt more strongly.

Positioning for Labor

- Changing positions during labor is a good way of easing discomfort and speeding up labor progress.
- Most favored positions include walking, rocking in a chair, squatting, and sitting on a birthing ball.
- The position chosen often depends on the comfort level and the stage of labor.

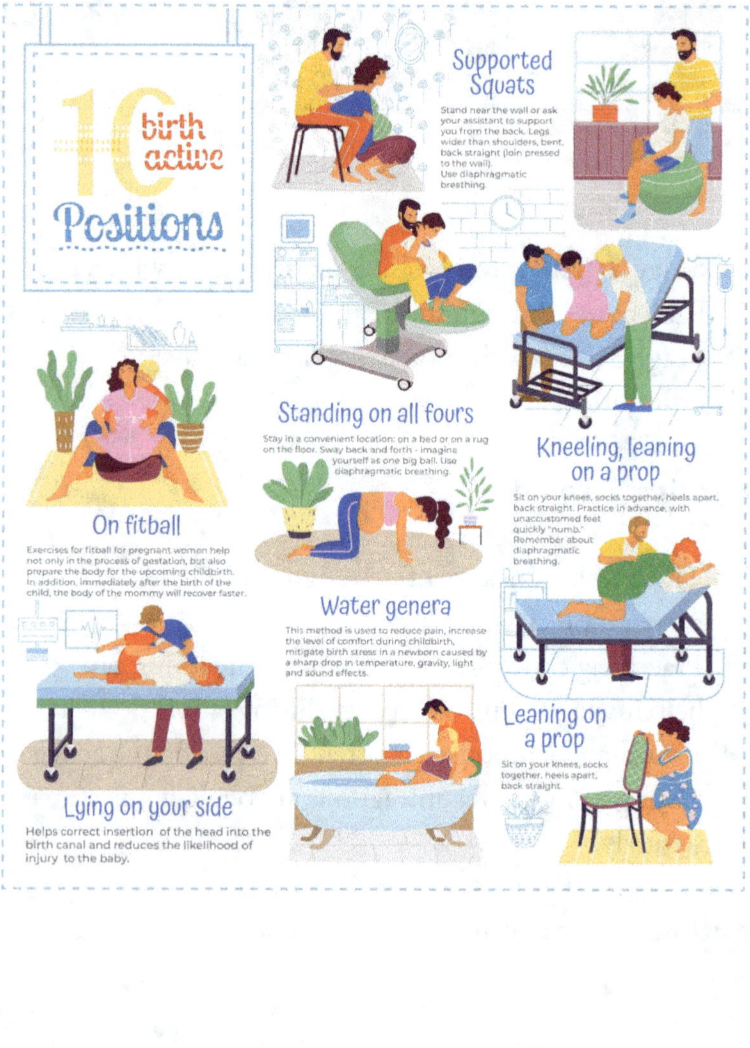
10 birth active Positions
Supported Squats
Stand near the wall or ask your assistant to support you from the back. Legs wider than shoulders, bent, back straight (loin pressed to the wall). Use diaphragmatic breathing.
Standing on all fours
Stay in a convenient location: on a bed or on a rug on the floor. Sway back and forth - imagine yourself as one big ball. Use diaphragmatic breathing.
Kneeling, leaning on a prop
Sit on your knees, socks together, heels apart, back straight. Practice in advance, with unaccustomed feet quickly "numb." Remember about diaphragmatic breathing.
On fitball
Exercises for fitball for pregnant women help not only in the process of gestation, but also prepare the body for the upcoming childbirth. In addition, immediately after the birth of the child, the body of the mommy will recover faster.
Water genera
This method is used to reduce pain, increase the level of comfort during childbirth, mitigate birth stress in a newborn caused by a sharp drop in temperature, gravity, light and sound effects.
Lying on your side
Helps correct insertion of the head into the birth canal and reduces the likelihood of injury to the baby.
Leaning on a prop
Sit on your knees, socks together, heels apart, back straight.

Electronic Fetal Monitoring (EFM)

- This is a common practice used at the time of labor to keep track of the baby's heart rate and the mother's contractions.
- EFM is accomplished by placing sensors on the mother's abdomen to monitor these vital signs.
- EFM helps healthcare providers to determine the well-being of the baby as labor progresses.

Fetal Blood Sampling

- Fetal blood sampling or fetal scalp blood sampling is the procedure used for checking the baby's oxygen levels during labor.
- A small blood sample is drawn from the baby's scalp through the cervix.
- This procedure is undertaken for immediate information about the baby's oxygen supply amidst concerns regarding the baby's well-being.

Bear in mind that every woman can have a unique labor experience and what has been provided is general guidance. It is always best to consult with your healthcare provider and gain personalized advice to address your specific concerns or questions regarding labor and childbirth.

14.10: Pain Management During Labor

Pain management during labor is an important aspect of childbirth and women have a range of options to help ease the discomfort and pain that accompanies labor contractions. The most commonly used techniques include epidurals, spinal blocks, and the use of Entonox (gas and air). Each of these options comes with its own set of pros, cons, side effects, and risks, and expectant moms should be well-informed about their options.

Epidural

Epidural anesthesia has proven to be a popular and highly effective pain management strategy during labor (*Pregnancy and birth*, 2018). It involves injecting medication into the epidural area of the spine, which numbs the lower half of the body, relieving labor pains while keeping the mother alert and conscious.

Pros

- **Effective pain relief:** Labor pains are considerably better managed with epidurals. They can help to ease contraction pain by blocking it from the waist down.
- **Allow for rest:** Epidurals enable the mother to rest if the labor is prolonged; this can be beneficial for both her and the baby.
- **Controlled dosage:** The epidural dosage can be modified to acquire the desired amount of pain reduction.

Cons

- **Limited mobility:** Epidurals can be problematic if the mother wants to move around during labor. This can stall labor, making it necessary to use interventions like Pitocin to speed up contractions.

- **Potential side effects:** These can include shivering, itching, and a drop in blood pressure.
- **Risk of complications:** There are some uncommon risks connected with epidurals, like infection, headache, or nerve damage.

Myths

According to a National Vital Statistics Report by Osterman and Martin, published in 2011, over 60% of women in labor choose some form of anesthesia to control pain during childbirth. The most prevalent choices among these alternatives encompass epidural administration, spinal anesthesia, or a blend of the two known as combined spinal-epidural anesthesia.

Nevertheless, numerous women harbor misunderstandings about epidurals, emphasizing concerns about persistent back pain to assertions of potential harm to the baby. Here is a list of some of these debunked myths.

- **Myth:** Epidurals result in the mother having permanent back pain or paralysis.

Serious epidural complications, like paralysis, are very rare. Some women may have brief lower back discomfort near the insertion site, but it is usually temporary. Evidence shows that when it comes to long-term low back pain, disability, and movement issues after childbirth, there is no significant difference between those who opt for epidurals and those who choose other forms of pain management (Howell et al., 2002).

- **Myth:** Epidurals are not safe for the baby.

According to the American Society of Anesthesiologists (ASA, 2014), no evidence exists to support such concerns. The amount of medication reaching the baby is too minimal to cause harm.

- **Myth:** An epidural could disturb the birth experience.

Epidurals neither cause grogginess nor do they make your legs completely numb. Normally, you can walk after the procedure (if hospital policy allows this). Epidurals ease your pain while maintaining your ability to move about and feel contractions (Hidaka & Callister, 2012).

- **Myth:** There's a limited timeframe for getting an epidural.

You can request an epidural at any time throughout labor; this can be in the beginning, middle, or toward the end. The timing is flexible and depends on your comfort and needs.

- **Myth:** Epidurals can delay labor or elevate the risk of a C-section.

Epidurals do not delay labor or raise the likelihood of a C-section. Other factors, such as the baby's size or issues of labor progression, are common reasons contributing to C-sections.

- **Myth:** Getting an epidural indicates weakness.

Pain tolerance is different for everyone and choosing pain relief during labor is a personal decision. It does not represent a woman's strength or determination.

Spinal Block

Spinal block is a quick and effective form of pain management during labor. Spinal blocks, as opposed to epidurals, deliver medication directly into the cerebrospinal fluid, resulting in almost instantaneous pain relief from the waist down.

Pros

- **Quick onset:** Spinal blocks provide fast-acting relief and are often used for cesarean sections or when immediate pain relief is required.
- **Highly effective:** Spinal blocks, just like epidurals, are effective pain blockers during labor.

Cons

- **Limited duration:** Spinal blocks typically offer pain relief for a shorter time period in comparison to epidurals.
- **Limited mobility:** Similar to epidurals, spinal blocks can restrict mobility during labor.

Contraindications

Spinal blocks are generally safe, but they are not recommended for women with certain medical conditions like allergies or bleeding disorders. Your healthcare provider will determine your specific case.

Entonox (Gas and Air)

Entonox, or gas and air, is a self-administered pain relief treatment used during labor. The patient inhales a mixture of nitrous oxide and oxygen through a mask or mouthpiece.

Pros

- **Quick relief:** When inhaled, Entonox provides almost instant pain relief.
- **Self-administered:** The laboring woman gets to control when and how much Entonox she inhales. This gives her a sense of control over pain management.

Cons

- **Limited effectiveness:** When compared to epidurals or spinal blocks, Entonox may not be as effective in providing total relief from pain.
- **Dizziness and nausea:** Some women may feel dizzy or nauseous when using Entonox.

It is crucial for expectant mothers to consult with their healthcare provider about what their preferences and concerns are in regard to pain management. This will help them make an informed decision that aligns with their individual needs and the details of their labor.

14.11: Cesarean Section

What Is a C-Section and When Is It Necessary?

A Cesarean section, or a C-section, is a medical surgery involving the delivery of a baby through an incision made in the mother's abdomen and uterus. C-sections are usually performed under the following conditions:

- **Medical complications:** Certain types of medical conditions make a vaginal birth risky for either the mother or the baby or, in some cases, both (Sung & Mahdy, 2023). Some examples may include placenta previa, certain heart conditions, or active genital herpes.
- **Fetal distress:** If continuous monitoring of the infant during labor reveals fetal distress or worries about the baby's well-being, a C-section may be needed to ensure safe delivery.
- **Breech presentation:** In cases where the baby is in a breech (bottom-first) or transverse (sideways) position close to the delivery time, a C-section is recommended to avoid complications.
- **Previous C-section:** If a woman has undergone a previous C-section, the safer option would be a repeat C-section instead of attempting a vaginal birth after cesarean (VBAC).

Benefits

- **Life-saving:** Sometimes, labor is riddled with complications and this is when C-sections can be life-saving for both the mother and the baby.
- **Controlled timing:** C-sections allow the birth to be scheduled, which can be beneficial in cases of medical emergency.
- **Reduced risk of birth injuries:** C-sections could minimize the risk of birth injuries, particularly in cases where the baby's size is too big for a vaginal birth or when there are issues with the birth canal.

Risks

- **Surgical complications:** C-sections, like any other surgical operations, are not without their share of inherent risks, consisting of infection, bleeding, and anesthesia problems.
- **Longer recovery:** Recovery time from a C-section is often longer than that from a vaginal birth and may also include postoperative pain and discomfort.
- **Future pregnancies:** C-sections can have an impact on future pregnancies, possibly enhancing the risk of uterine rupture or placenta accreta.

Recovery Guide and Recommendations After a C-Section

- **Pain management:** Prescriptions given to you by your healthcare provider can help in dealing with post-operative pain. Follow the recommended dosage and schedule.

- **Rest and activity:** At first, rest is important to help with healing. Gradually, undertake light, low-impact activities as advised by your healthcare provider to prevent complications.
- **Incision care:** Ensure that the incision is always clean and dry. Look out for signs of infection, such as redness, swelling, or discharge, and contact your healthcare provider if you see any.
- **Emotional support:** Emotional recovery is just as important as physical recovery. Emotional support from loved ones, support groups, or a mental health professional can all be a great source of recuperation.
- **Breastfeeding:** This is possible after a C-section if the mother wishes to breastfeed.

This marks the culmination of your journey from pregnancy to labor. The next part explores valuable insights into the various aspects of post-delivery issues, ranging from physical recovery to emotional well-being and newborn care.

Part Four

Birthing—Welcome Baby!

Giving birth should be your greatest achievement, not your greatest fear.

—Jane Weideman

Chapter 15

Delivery

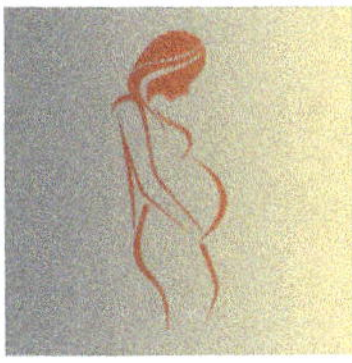

The delivery process is a crucial stage in childbirth, including various techniques and procedures to ensure a newborn's safe arrival. This chapter provides insights into the different aspects of delivery, from natural vaginal deliveries to more specialized techniques, along with critical post-delivery considerations.

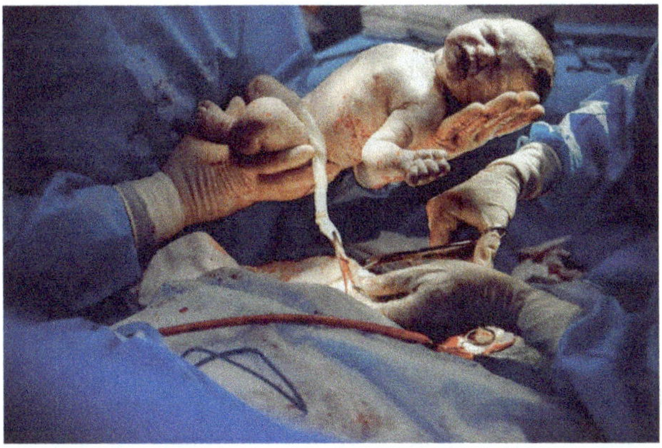

15.1: Delivery Process

The delivery process is an important milestone in childbirth and consists of several crucial elements:

- **Natural vaginal delivery:** This is the most common method of childbirth. The process involves the baby being born through the mother's birth canal with the natural progression of labor, contractions, and the eventual appearance of the baby's head and body. If there are no complications, this is the most favorable option.
- **Episiotomy:** This procedure involves making a surgical cut in the perineum, the area between the vaginal opening and the anus, at the time of childbirth. It is done to widen the vaginal opening and thereby enabling a smoother delivery. Episiotomies are often resorted to if there is a risk of severe tearing or if a fast delivery is required for the sake of the baby's well-being.
- **Indications for getting an episiotomy:** The need for an episiotomy arises in cases where the baby is in distress, there are baby position complications (like breech), for premature births, the baby size is larger than normal, there is a need for forceps or vacuum delivery, or if there is a danger of severe tearing during delivery (Choudhari et al., 2022).
- **Post-episiotomy pain management with medication:** It is normal for women to feel pain and discomfort after having endured an episiotomy. To help handle this kind of discomfort, pain

medications like over-the-counter pain relievers or prescribed analgesics can be used to gain a more comfortable recovery.

- **Sitz bath for managing episiotomy pain and discomfort:** A good way of easing pain and encouraging healing after an episiotomy is having a sitz bath. This involves dipping the perineal area in warm water; this will reduce swelling and provide soothing relief.
- **Post-episiotomy infection prevention tips:** After the episiotomy, it is essential that the incision be kept clean and dry, sanitary pads are regularly changed, and proper hygiene is practiced to avoid infection.
- **Post-episiotomy pain management:** Apart from medication and sitz baths, you can also deal with the pain by using cold packs to lessen swelling and discomfort. Adopt a gentle, gradual approach to returning to normal life activities.
- **First post-episiotomy bowel movement:** This can be very worrisome due to the potential for pain and discomfort. The situation can be overcome by staying hydrated, eating a high-fiber diet, and using stool softeners recommended by a healthcare provider.

15.2: Delivery Methods

Delivery methods involve various techniques used in obstetrics to help with childbirth if needed. The methods are resorted to when there are worries regarding the safety of the baby or mother during a natural delivery.

Forceps Birth

- **When needed:** The need for forceps arises when the baby's head is not descending properly through the birth canal, there are concerns about the baby's health, or when the mother is weary and unable to push effectively.
- **Risks:** Forceps delivery can have risks like potential injury to the baby's head or face, and there also exists the chance of tears or trauma to the mother's perineum. To mitigate these risks, careful monitoring and proper skill in the use of forceps are essential.

Ventouse Birth

- **When needed:** Ventouse or vacuum extraction using a soft cup is often used when a less invasive intervention than that of forceps is required or when the baby's head is not coming out as expected.
- **Risks:** Ventouse births can cause mild scalp injuries or, in rare cases, internal bleeding in the baby's head. To avoid complications, skillful application and monitoring of the vacuum are essential (Ali & Norwitz, 2009).

Healthcare experts carefully decide whether to use forceps or ventouse during delivery, based on the individual circumstances of the pregnancy and the well-being of both the mother and the baby. The healthcare team present must have adequate skill and experience to undertake these procedures safely and successfully while minimizing potential risks.

15.3: Birthing the Placenta

This is the process of delivering the placenta after childbirth, and in recent times, a new trend has evolved of exploring novel uses of the placenta, such as consuming it in different forms to potentially cure postpartum depression (PPD). This method includes either boiling and consuming the placenta or drying and grinding it for oral powder pills. However, it is important to recognize that the scientific data supporting these claims is limited and placenta encapsulation carries substantial risks.

Why Do People Eat Their Placenta?

Fans of placenta consumption highlight a variety of benefits, including prevention of anemia, increased milk production, hormone balance, and reduced risk of PPD. However, these supposed advantages are mostly based on anecdotal evidence, and there is a notable absence of robust scientific support (Hayes, 2016).

What Are the Benefits of Eating the Placenta?

Scientific evidence on how placenta consumption in humans can be beneficial is limited. Small studies have revealed possible links to increased breast milk supply and pain relief, though this observation was made in rats, not humans. Moreover, the risks of consuming human tissue, such as the placenta, have not been extensively researched (Mota-Rojas et al., 2020).

Placenta Encapsulation: What You Need to Know

Placenta encapsulation is a trend where the placenta, the organ responsible for feeding a growing baby throughout pregnancy, is turned into pills after delivery. People do this with the belief that it can help with postpartum depression (PPD) and overall health.

Mainstream Medical Viewpoint

Most mainstream medical experts stress that there is no scientific evidence to support eating of the placenta. Large-scale studies have failed to prove its benefits, and there are worries regarding the potential risks of this treatment (Cleveland Clinic, 2019).

Warnings and Health Concerns

The Centers for Disease Control and Prevention (CDC) strongly discourages the practice. A report was released highlighting a sad incident in which a mother transferred a recurrent Group B Streptococcus infection to her baby because of consuming her own placenta capsules, underscoring the possible risks involved with this trend (Buser et al., 2017).

What to Do If You Decide to Eat the Placenta Despite Risks

If you still want to try placenta encapsulation, here are some precautions to consider:

- **Check with your hospital or birthing center:** Placentas are often treated as medical waste in hospitals. If you want to keep it, you'll need to make plans ahead of time. Check with your healthcare provider to ensure compatibility with their policies.
- **Professional preparation:** Consider hiring professional placenta encapsulation services. The placenta is dried, powdered, and encapsulated in this

process to make it easier to swallow. However, the CDC warns that safety and efficacy criteria for placenta sterilization and processing are insufficient.

- **Follow safe-prep practices:** If you would like to prepare the placenta at home, make sure you follow safe guidelines. You can gain information about DIY supplies, kits, and instructions on the internet. To prevent spoilage, properly preserve or cook the placenta. Some people choose to hire professional placenta preparers or midwives to handle the processing.
- **Monitoring and caution:** If, after having taken placenta pills or eaten cooked placenta, you experience any adverse reactions or illness, stop immediately. In cases of suspected PPD, do not just depend on placenta consumption; promptly consult your healthcare provider for appropriate treatment and get the proper therapy or medication.

In the end, while some women may decide to try placenta encapsulation, it is important to make informed decisions, prioritize safety, and pursue evidence-based care for post-partum health and happiness.

15.4: Retained Placental Complications

Retained placental complications arise in situations where part or all of the placenta or fetal membranes are still within the uterus following childbirth, instead of being fully removed as part of the normal birthing process. This condition can cause a whole range of serious health problems for the mother, requiring immediate medical assistance (Perlman & Carusi, 2019).

Causes of Retained Placenta

- **Incomplete separation:** Occasionally, the placenta may not fully separate from the uterine wall, preventing its complete removal.
- **Placenta adherence:** Placenta accreta, increta, or percreta are conditions where the placenta abnormally clings to the uterine wall, making removal difficult.
- **Uterine atony:** This is when the uterus fails to contract properly after delivery, preventing the placenta from being expelled.

Complications and Risks

- **Postpartum hemorrhage (PPH):** Retained placental tissue is a medical emergency as it can cause serious bleeding. PPH can lead to a fall in blood pressure, anemia, and shock, all of which can be fatal.
- **Infection:** The presence of retained placental tissue can enhance the risk of uterine infection, manifesting with symptoms like fever, pain, and abnormal discharge.
- **Delayed healing:** Due to retained placental fragments, the uterus may not contract properly or heal as expected. This can possibly result in prolonged recovery and discomfort for the mother.

- **Uterine rupture:** In rare cases, the uterus can end up rupturing because of the pressure generated by retained placental tissue. This situation is urgent and calls for surgery without delay.

Diagnosis usually consists of a physical examination, ultrasound, and monitoring of symptoms. Management options may include

- **Manual removal:** Under sterile conditions, healthcare providers may manually extract the residual placental tissue with their hands or instruments, usually under anesthesia.
- **Medication:** Oxytocin or prostaglandins are typical medications to help the uterus contract and expel the tissue.
- **Dilation and Curettage (D&C):** This is a surgical procedure involving the dilation of the cervix to enable the scraping or suctioning of tissue from the uterus.
- **Hysterectomy:** In extreme cases or when other treatments fail, a hysterectomy (removal of the uterus) may be the only alternative.

Early identification and intervention are crucial to avoid complications connected with retained placental tissue. Mothers who have postpartum bleeding, chronic pain, or signs of infection after delivery should seek immediate medical help to ensure their well-being and avert future health problems.

15.5: Apgar Score—Normal Versus Abnormal Score

The Apgar Score is a quick and easy examination performed by healthcare professionals to determine a newborn's overall health and well-being soon after birth. The Apgar Score, named after Dr. Virginia Apgar, who established it in the 1950s, offers a snapshot of the baby's condition at one minute and five minutes after birth. It is made up of five important criteria, each of which is rated on a scale of 0 to 2, with a total score of 10. These are the criteria:

- **Appearance (skin color):** This criterion examines the baby's skin color, where a score of 2 indicates a baby with a pink or rosy complexion, a score of 1 indicates a baby with a bluish or pale look, and a score of 0 indicates a newborn who appears blue or gray all over.
- **Pulse rate (heart rate):** The heart rate measures how well the baby's heart is working. A heart rate of more than 100 beats per minute gets a score of 2, a heart rate of less than 100 beats per minute gets a score of 1, and no detectable heart rate gets a score of 0.
- **Grimace response (reflexes):** This evaluates the baby's reflexes and response to stimuli, such as a light pinch or stimulation of the sole of the foot. A score of 2 is assigned for a forceful response, a score of 1 for a weak response, and a score of 0 for no response.
- **Activity (muscle tone):** Muscle tone represents the baby's overall muscle strength and activity level. A score of 2 indicates active and strong muscle tone, 1

for some muscle limpness, and 0 for fully limp muscles.

- **Respiration (breathing):** This criterion assesses the baby's breathing effort. A score of 2 represents strong and regular breathing, 1 for irregular or slow breathing, and 0 for no breathing at all.

Normal Apgar Score

- A total Apgar Score of 7 to 10 at one minute after birth is considered normal.
- A baby with a normal Apgar Score is normally pink, depicts a heart rate of over 100 beats per minute, responds to stimuli with crying or active movements, has strong muscle tone, and regular breathing.

Abnormal Apgar Score

- An Apgar Score of less than 7 at one minute after birth may signal that the baby needs medical intervention or extra monitoring.
- A low Apgar Score may indicate the presence of potentially serious concerns like respiratory distress, heart defects, or delivery complications.

The Apgar Score is recalculated five minutes after birth to measure the baby's response to any interventions or resuscitation efforts. This gives a deeper understanding of the baby's condition and helps guide further medical decisions and care.

15.6: Newborn Screen (NBS)—Normal Versus Abnormal Results

Newborn screening is a vital aspect of pediatric healthcare that aims to detect potential health problems in infants soon after birth.

Normal Results

A normal NBS result usually indicates that examinations of a newborn's blood or other biological samples did not reveal any worrisome medical issues at the time of testing. It has the following benefits:

- **Relief and reassurance:** Normal NBS findings reassure parents and healthcare providers that the baby does not seem to have any of the major congenital or metabolic diseases screened for in the test panel at this time.
- **Early intervention:** While normal NBS results are comforting, it is important to note that they do not represent a lifetime of perfect health. Instead, they give a chance for early intervention in case any issues do emerge later in a child's development, as many illnesses can present symptoms well after the neonatal period.

Abnormal Results

An abnormal NBS result manifests that the screening tests have identified markers or levels suggesting the presence of certain congenital or metabolic disorders. If your newborn's

NBS results come back as abnormal, here is what you should be aware of:

- **Further testing required:** An abnormal result is not necessarily a confirmation of the presence of a disorder, but rather signals a need for additional diagnostic tests to verify or rule out the condition. These follow-up tests are necessary for acquiring an accurate diagnosis.
- **Early intervention and treatment:** Early detection of disorders through NBS enables quick medical intervention and treatment when necessary. Timely intervention can considerably improve the outcomes for many conditions screened for in the NBS panel.
- **Emotional impact:** Receiving abnormal NBS results can be tough to deal with for parents. It is essential to get help from healthcare professionals and support groups to understand the diagnostic process and make informed decisions about your child's health.
- **Education and counseling:** Healthcare providers are there to help parents properly understand the condition, treatment options, and available resources. This support can help parents make informed decisions and obtain appropriate care for their child.
- **Family screening:** In cases where a genetic disorder definitely exists, families may be recommended to seek genetic counseling and testing in order to better understand the genetic basis of the condition and

determine the risk of having another affected child in the future.

In conclusion, newborn screening is vital for identifying possible health problems in babies and also enables early intervention and treatment when necessary. Both normal and abnormal results are useful in guiding parents and healthcare providers in providing the best possible care for newborns.

15.7: Neonatal Jaundice

Neonatal jaundice, or neonatal hyperbilirubinemia, is an often occurring condition in newborns that causes the skin and whites of the eyes to turn yellow. It develops due to an excess buildup of bilirubin, a yellow pigment generated during the breakdown of red blood cells, in a baby's bloodstream. Neonatal jaundice commonly affects up to 60% of all full-term newborns and 80% of premature babies in the first week following birth (Ansong-Assoku et al., 2023).

Causes

Neonatal jaundice is the result of a newborn's liver not being fully developed yet and, thus, has difficulty processing bilirubin effectively. There are several possible reasons why bilirubin levels elevate in newborns, including

- **Physiological jaundice:** This is the most common type of neonatal jaundice and makes an appearance normally within the first few days of life. It usually lasts for a short period and is a benign condition caused by the baby's underdeveloped liver and enhanced breakdown of fetal red blood cells.

- **Breastfeeding jaundice:** Inadequate breastfeeding, mostly because of latch issues, infrequent feeding, or not enough milk supply, can cause dehydration. A drop in the baby's urine output can lead to increased bilirubin levels as it is excreted through urine. Providing proper breastfeeding support and hydration is essential.
- **Breast milk jaundice:** This is caused by certain substances in breast milk interfering with the baby's ability to process bilirubin. It normally appears after the first week of life and can last for several weeks.
- **Blood type incompatibility:** If the mother and baby have different blood types (e.g., Rh or ABO incompatibility), the newborn's immune system may break down red blood cells at a faster rate, resulting in higher bilirubin levels.

Symptoms

The yellowing of the skin and eyes (icterus) is the most visible symptom of neonatal jaundice. In more extreme cases, the baby may seem lethargic, feed poorly, or cry loudly. Occasionally, extremely high bilirubin levels can result in kernicterus, a disorder that can cause permanent neurological damage (NHS, 2022a).

Treatment

The cause and severity of the illness determine the treatment for neonatal jaundice. Common treatment options include the following:

- **Phototherapy:** The most widely used treatment in which the baby is exposed to special blue or white lights that aid in the breakdown of bilirubin in the skin. The baby's eyes are normally covered to shield them from the light.
- **Exchange transfusion:** In more severe cases of jaundice or when other treatments have failed, it may be necessary to undertake a partial or complete exchange transfusion. This involves replacing the baby's blood with fresh donor blood to lower bilirubin levels.
- **Feeding support:** In cases of breastfeeding jaundice, ensuring that the baby is nursing properly or providing alternative feeding methods for gaining adequate nutrition can help cure the condition.
- **Treatment of underlying causes:** If the illness is caused by underlying medical conditions like blood type incompatibility, those conditions may need to be remedied.

It is important for parents to seek medical attention if they notice jaundice in their newborn. Early diagnosis and proper treatment are essential to avoid complications and safeguard the baby's health. Pediatricians and neonatologists are fully equipped to manage and treat neonatal jaundice.

15.8: Stillbirth and Dealing With the Loss of a Baby

Stillbirth is the devastating event of a baby being born with no signs of life after the 20th week of pregnancy. It is a heart-breaking loss for parents and their families who are waiting for the arrival of a healthy baby but, instead, have to bear the loss of their child before or during childbirth. Stillbirth is often discernable from miscarriage, which usually happens before the 20th week of pregnancy.

Causes

- **Placental problems:** Issues like placental abruption (when the placenta prematurely separates from the uterine wall) or placental insufficiency (when the placenta does not supply enough oxygen and nutrients to the baby) can result in stillbirth.
- **Infections:** Incurring infections like cytomegalovirus (CMV) or listeria during pregnancy, can endanger the growing baby and may cause stillbirth.
- **Genetic factors:** Genetic defects in the baby can lead to stillbirth.
- **Chronic medical conditions:** Diabetes, high blood pressure, and certain autoimmune illnesses can all elevate the chance of stillbirth if not properly treated during pregnancy.
- **Umbilical cord issues:** These include problems like cord compression or an actual knot in the cord, which can limit the flow of blood to the baby.
- **Fetal growth restriction:** Sometimes, the baby is just not growing properly in the womb, resulting in stillbirth.
- **Maternal health issues:** If the mother is not well or has an illness like preeclampsia, it can affect the baby's well-being and cause stillbirth.

- **Environmental factors:** Being exposed to environmental toxins or consuming certain medications during pregnancy can also be linked with stillbirth.

Celebrities and Icons Who Have Shared Their Loss Publicly

Chrissy Teigen is one of many celebrities who chose to openly share her experience of stillbirth. In September 2020, she and her husband, John Legend, told the heartbreaking story of how they lost their baby boy, whom they had already named Jack. Chrissy Teigen shared the sad moments, including intimate photographs from the hospital, on social media. She received immense support from fans and fellow celebrities for her openness in such a difficult time.

Christina Perri, the famous singer-songwriter, shared her sad experience of stillbirth on Twitter in November 2020. She and her husband, Paul Costabile, announced their daughter died in the third trimester of pregnancy. Perri was honest with her fans, posting a moving photo of herself and Costabile holding the hand of their stillborn child. She had previously said that her pregnancy was in peril and that she had been hospitalized for close monitoring. She had already been through a miscarriage before in January 2020. Christina Perri and her husband have two daughters.

Michelle Obama, the former First Lady, shared deeply personal details in her memoir *Becoming*, released in November 2018, about her struggles with fertility and pregnancy loss. She disclosed that she had struggled to get pregnant and had suffered a miscarriage. Michelle Obama described the event as leaving her feeling inadequate, bewildered, and alone. She also mentioned the use of IVF treatments to conceive their two daughters, Sasha and Malia. During promotion interviews for her book, Michelle stressed the importance of discussing the truth about women's bodies and fertility issues, encouraging open conversations about these matters among women.

Celebrity stories of pregnancy loss and fertility struggles have inspired important conversations about the difficulties that many families face. Now, it is time to move from the anticipation of new life to the crucial journey of postpartum and newborn care, emphasizing the well-being of both mother and baby.

Part Five

The "Fourth Trimester"— Postpartum and Newborn Care

When he finally was placed into my arms, I looked into his precious eyes and felt an overwhelming, unconditional love; I never felt so complete and empowered in my life.

— Gisele Bündchen

Chapter 16

"Homing" and Bonding With Baby

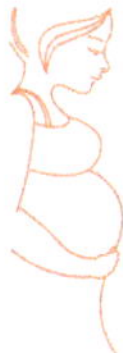

When your baby is born, not only does this mark the end of pregnancy, but also the beginning of a new adventure. The first three months of your newborn's life outside the womb are commonly known as the "fourth trimester." Creating a strong link with your infant is critical during this period, and a concept known as "homing" might help make this transition easier.

What Is "Homing"?

"Homing" is the preparation of a cozy and safe space at home, enabling your baby to feel as comfortable as they did in the womb. So

- **Set up a cozy spot:** Ensure your baby's nursery or sleeping area has a comfy crib, soft blankets, and a soothing atmosphere.
- **Mimic the womb:** Try techniques like swaddling (wrapping your baby snugly in a blanket), using

white noise machines, and sticking to a consistent schedule for feeding, diaper changes, and sleep.

Building a Strong Bond With Your Baby

Bonding with your baby is all about building a loving and secure connection. Here's how to do this:

- **Skin-to-skin contact:** Holding your baby against your bare skin not only provides warmth but is also a great way to connect emotionally.
- **Talk and make eye contact:** Even though your baby at present is too young to understand what you are saying, talking to them in a soothing tone while looking at them helps them feel close to you.
- **Cuddling:** Snuggle your baby from time to time, like during feeding, diaper changes, or just because it is a great way to bond.

Emotional Connection

Understanding your baby's behaviors and being there for them is crucial for bonding.

- **Read the signals:** Learn to recognize your baby's cries, body movements, and facial expressions. Giving them prompt responses helps to make them feel safer.
- **Be emotionally available:** Demonstrate to your baby that you're there for them emotionally. When they are upset or in need of consolation, console them. This fosters attachment and trust.

Taking Care of Yourself

Remember, to be the best parent, your own care cannot be ignored. Looking after a newborn can be exhausting. Make sure you are getting enough rest, reach out to friends and family for help, and learn to manage your stress.

Family Bonding

Involving other family members is also important. So, include everyone! Or just those who would truly like to. Even though the baby is your precious bundle of joy, encourage your partner, grandparents, and siblings to bond with the baby too. This is not only beneficial for your baby but also strengthens the family bond.

16.1: Before Leaving the Hospital: Birth Certificate; Car Seat, Welcome Home Events/Parties

Before you are ready to depart the hospital with your little bundle of joy, make sure that you have everything right and ready for a safe and smooth transition home. Here are some important considerations:

- **Birth certificate:** Ensure you have a copy of your baby's birth certificate. This document is required for a variety of purposes, including getting identification and applying for government benefits.
- **Car seat:** A properly installed car seat is a must for safely transporting your baby home. Make sure you have the correct car seat for your child's age, weight, and height, and that it is placed correctly in your vehicle. Most medical facilities will not let you leave

until you have confirmed that you have a suitable car seat.

- **Welcome home events/parties:** If you're looking forward to having welcome home festivities or parties, remember your baby's safety comes first. Therefore, you should
- Put a limit on the number of guests, especially during the first few weeks when your baby's immune system is still developing.
- Prevent infection risks by asking guests to wash their hands before they hold the baby.
- Arrange for a designated, safe space for your baby. This will help keep the baby calm during the event, away from excessive noise and potential hazards.
- **Babyproof your home:** It is essential to have your living space babyproofed before bringing your baby home. Here is how this can be done:
- Install safety gates at the top and bottom of stairs.
- Cover electrical outlets.
- Secure heavy furniture and potentially dangerous objects.
- Small objects that can cause choking hazards should be kept out of reach.
- Lock cabinets to keep harmful substances and objects out of reach.

16.2: Breast Milk Versus Formula

Breast milk and formula are two available options for feeding infants; each has its own set of advantages and considerations.

Here are some details on the differences between breastmilk and formula:

Source

- **Breast milk:** Breast milk is natural milk that a mother's body produces in response to her baby's needs. It is a living fluid with a unique blend of nutrients, antibodies, and immune-boosting properties that aid in safeguarding the baby from infections and illnesses. Breast milk adapts to the baby's changing nutritional needs as they grow.
- **Formula:** This is a commercially manufactured substitute for breast milk. It is prepared by combining ingredients to replicate the nutritional content of breast milk. Formula is not a living substance and it lacks the immune-boosting properties of breast milk.

Nutritional Content

- **Breast milk:** This milk naturally meets the specific needs of the baby. It has an ideal balance of carbohydrates, proteins, fats, vitamins, and minerals, along with antibodies, enzymes, and growth factors that aid in a newborn's development.
- **Formula:** Even though infant formula attempts to mimic breast milk, being carefully formulated to supply necessary nutrients for a baby's growth and development, it may not have the same composition or immune-boosting properties.

Convenience

- **Breast milk:** When it comes to accessibility and temperature, breastfeeding can be more convenient. Breast milk is always ready and at the correct temperature, and it does not need to be prepared or sterilized.
- **Formula:** Formula feeding is a good alternative in situations where parents desire a flexible schedule or when the mother is unable to breastfeed. In the case of formula milk, it requires preparation, doing things like measuring, mixing, and sterilizing bottles and equipment.

Availability

- **Breast milk:** As long as the mother is capable, and chooses to do so, breast milk is readily available. It is free and has a low impact on the environment.
- **Formula:** Formula has to be bought and does not rely on the mother's ability to produce milk. Furthermore, it might be costly over time.

Health Benefits

- **Breast milk:** There are various health benefits of breastfeeding for both the baby and the mother. It can help protect the newborn from infections, lower the chance of allergies, and enhance mother-baby bonding. Breastfeeding can also provide certain health benefits to the mother, including lowering the

risk of certain cancers and assisting with postpartum recovery.
- **Formula:** Formula provides necessary nutrition for babies who cannot or do not receive breast milk. It is a viable option in cases where breastfeeding is not possible or chosen.

Special Considerations

- Breastfeeding is not always possible for all mothers due to medical or personal reasons. In such cases, formula feeding becomes the key option for baby nutrition.
- To provide flexibility and fulfill their baby's requirements, some moms prefer to combine breastfeeding and formula feeding. This is known as mixed feeding.

In the end, the choice between breast milk and formula is based on individual circumstances, such as the mother's health, lifestyle, and personal preferences. Consult with a healthcare provider to make an informed decision that best meets the needs of both the baby and the mother. Breast milk and formula can both be healthy and effective ways to nourish and nurture a newborn.

16.3: Feeding and Bonding: Breastfeeding Versus Formula feeding

Feeding and bonding with your baby is an important aspect of their physical and emotional development. Both breastfeeding and formula feeding provide unique opportunities for bonding, but they differ in terms of dynamics and effects on the parent-child relationship:

Breastfeeding

- **Physical bonding:** Breastfeeding enables intimate physical contact between the mother (or primary caregiver) and the baby. During nursing, skin-to-skin contact releases oxytocin, also known as the "love hormone," which fosters a strong emotional connection.
- **Biological connection:** Breast milk naturally meets the nutritional needs of a baby and contains antibodies that help boost the infant's immune system. Breastfeeding strengthens the biological bond between mother and baby, as the mother's body responds to the baby's cues like hunger and comfort.
- **Responsive parenting:** Breastfeeding often involves on-demand feeding, allowing parents to respond quickly to the baby's hunger and comfort needs. This attentiveness can help deepen the bond by strengthening the baby's trust and sense of security.
- **Challenges and stress:** While breastfeeding can be a beautiful bonding experience, it can also come with repercussions like latch issues, nipple soreness, and milk supply concerns, creating stress for some parents. Seeking advice and support from lactation consultants or healthcare experts can help you overcome these difficulties.

Formula Feeding

- **Shared responsibility:** Formula feeding enables parents and caregivers to participate in feeding and looking after the baby. This promotes sharing responsibilities for the baby's care. This can help strengthen the bond between the baby and multiple caregivers.
- **Predictable schedules:** Formula feeding often has a more predictable schedule because it takes longer to digest than breast milk. This predictability can help parents develop routines and plan their daily activities more easily.
- **Bonding opportunities:** While formula feeding lacks the physical act of nursing, there are still many bonding opportunities during feeding. Holding, caressing, and maintaining eye contact with the baby while bottle-feeding can form an emotional bond.
- **Flexibility:** Formula feeding can offer more control over when and how often your baby is fed, giving the advantage of being able to share feeding duties with others. This is especially beneficial for working parents or families with hectic schedules.

It is worth mentioning that bonding with a baby does not entirely depend on the feeding method. Bonding can occur through a variety of interactions, such as playtime, soothing, talking, and simply being present for the baby's needs. Every family has its own unique situation, and the choice between breastfeeding and formula feeding should take into account the parents' preferences, circumstances, and the baby's needs (Radzyminski & Callister, 2016).

Furthermore, the important point is to provide a loving and nurturing environment for the baby, regardless of the feeding method chosen. Both breastfeeding and formula feeding can be strong bonding experiences when done with love and care.

16.4: Burping and Colic

Burping

Babies burp frequently during and after feedings. It is important to help your baby expel air that they may have swallowed while nursing. Burping is necessary because trapped air in the stomach can cause pain and lead to fussiness or colic. Here are some more details on burping.

Why Burping Is Necessary

- Babies, whether breastfed or bottle-fed, have a tendency to swallow air while eating. This trapped air might cause gas in their tummies, making them uncomfortable.
- Burping helps release the trapped air, relieving gassiness and pain.

When to Burp Your Baby

- Bottle-fed babies can be made to burp every 2–3 ounces during feeding.
- For breastfed babies, burping can be done when switching breasts or midway through a feeding.

How to Burp Your Baby

- Burping a baby can be done in numerous ways, including over the shoulder, sitting on your lap, or holding the baby upright. Experiment to find what works best for your baby.
- Pat or rub your baby's back gently until you hear or feel a burp. Be patient, as this process may require a few minutes.

Although some newborns may not need to burp after every feeding, it is still a good practice to try.

Colic

Colic is a term that refers to excessive, often unpredictable crying in an otherwise healthy and well-fed infant. Colic is most common in babies under three months old and can be extremely distressing for both the baby and the parents. Here is more information about colic.

Characteristics of Colic

- Colic is characterized when an otherwise healthy baby is crying for at least three hours a day, for three days a week, for three weeks or more (Cleveland Clinic, 2023f).
- Crying is most common in the late afternoon or evening.
- During episodes of crying, colicky babies may clench their fists, arch their backs, and have a firm, bloated abdomen.

Possible Causes of Colic

- What exactly causes colic is not really known and may be due to multiple factors, including gastrointestinal discomfort, developing digestive systems, and sensitivity to stimuli.
- Colic is not caused by the parents doing something wrong, and it often resolves on its own by 3 to 4 months of age.

Coping With Colic

- If you feel your baby has colic, you should see a pediatrician to rule out any underlying medical problems.
- Swaddling, gentle rocking, using white noise machines, providing a pacifier, and ensuring that your baby has been properly fed and changed are all ways of coping with colic.
- Taking turns with a partner or requesting help from friends and family can help you cope with the stress of a colicky infant.

Keep in mind that each infant is different and may require different approaches to deal with the issue. If you're worried about your baby's crying or behavior, it is always a good idea to get advice and assistance from your pediatrician.

16.5: Care of the Umbilical Cord Stump

Caring for the umbilical cord stump is a key part of newborn care. This is the small, usually whitish, or yellowish remnant of the umbilical cord that remains connected to the baby's belly button after birth. Proper care helps in preventing infection and ensures a safe healing process. Here is how to care for the umbilical cord stump:

Keep It Clean and Dry

- Gently clean the cord stump's base with warm water and mild soap once a day, typically during the baby's bath time. Clean around the base with a soft, clean cloth or cotton ball.
- After cleaning, make sure the cord stump is totally dry. You can gently pat it dry with a soft, clean cloth.

Avoid Immersion in Water

- While giving your newborn a sponge wash is acceptable, avoid immersing the baby in water until the umbilical cord stump has fallen off. Keeping it dry helps it to heal faster.

Use Fold-Down Diapers

- Keep the area around the cord stump dry by folding down the top of your baby's diaper. This will expose the stump and allow air to circulate around it, helping to dry it out.

Avoid Tight Clothing

- To avoid friction and irritation around the cord stump, dress your baby in loose-fitting clothing.

Watch for Signs of Infection

- Keep an eye out for signs of infection such as redness, warmth, swelling, discharge (particularly if it's pus-like or foul-smelling), or if your baby seems unusually irritable or uncomfortable.
- If you observe any of these symptoms, contact your pediatrician immediately, as this could indicate an infection that requires medical attention.

Let It Fall Off Naturally

- The umbilical cord stump normally falls off on its own one to three weeks after birth. Do not try to pull it off prematurely, even if it looks like it is hanging by a thread. Let it detach naturally to reduce the risk of infection.

Don't Use Alcohol or Ointments

- It is no longer advisable to apply alcohol or ointments on the umbilical cord stump unless specifically advised to do so by your healthcare provider (Cleveland Clinic, 2022f). Keeping it clean and dry is usually enough.

Practice Good Hand Hygiene

- Always wash your hands properly before and after touching the cord stump or caring for your baby. This aids in preventing the spread of germs and lowers the risk of infection.

Caring for the umbilical cord stump is a simple yet crucial element of newborn care. It is essential to be patient and careful in maintaining hygiene and looking for signs of infection until the stump detaches naturally. If you have any concerns or questions concerning your baby's umbilical cord care, don't hesitate to consult your pediatrician or healthcare provider for guidance.

16.6: Diaper Changing and Baby's First Bath

As a new parent, you'll need to do basic duties such as diaper changing and giving your baby their first bath. Here is an elaboration on both of these activities.

Diaper Changing

Before you begin, gather all of the required items, such as clean diapers, wipes, diaper rash cream, a changing pad, and a change of clothes for your baby. Keeping everything within arm's reach keeps you organized and prevents you from leaving your baby unattended.

- **Choose a safe location:** Find a flat, secure surface for diaper changes. Most parents use a changing table, but a clean, soft area on the floor with a changing mat can also be used.

- **Wash hands:** To avoid the spread of germs, always thoroughly wash your hands with soap and water before changing your baby's diaper.
- **Be prepared:** Lay your baby on their back on the changing mat and unfasten the dirty diaper. Wipe away as much of the mess as possible with the front of the diaper.
- **Cleanse gently:** Use baby wipes or a moist cloth to properly clean your baby's bottom. Cleaning in the creases and folds is important but avoid excessive rubbing because a baby's skin is delicate and sensitive. Allow the area to air dry or pat dry with a clean cloth.
- **Apply diaper cream (if needed):** If your baby's bottom has signs of diaper rash or irritation, apply a diaper rash cream or ointment as recommended by your pediatrician.
- **Secure a fresh diaper:** Gently lift your baby's legs and put a clean diaper under them. Secure the diaper firmly, striking a balance between ensuring it is snug and comfortable without being overly tight.
- **Dispose of the dirty diaper properly:** Roll up the dirty diaper, fasten it with the tabs, and discard it in a diaper pail or lidded trash can. After handling the used diaper, wash your hands again.

Baby's First Bath

- **Timing:** You do not have to give your baby a full bath right after birth. Initially, sponge baths are advised until the umbilical cord stump falls off (normally within the first few weeks). Following that, you can progress to a gentle baby tub bath.

- **Gather supplies:** Gather all of the necessary bath items, including a baby tub, mild baby soap, a soft washcloth, baby shampoo (if necessary), a clean towel, and clean baby clothes.
- **Fill the tub:** If using a baby tub, fill it with a few inches of lukewarm water. Test the water temperature by dipping your elbow in it. Ensure it is comfortably warm but not hot.
- **Undress your baby:** Gently remove your baby's clothing but keep them wrapped in a towel so that they do not get too cold.
- **Support the head:** Lower your baby into the tub while holding them securely, taking care to support their head and neck.
- **Gentle cleansing:** Gently cleanse your baby's body with a soft washcloth and mild baby soap. Take extra care around the eyes, ears, and genitals.
- **Rinse and dry:** Rinse your baby thoroughly with clean water using a cup or your hand. Lift them out of the tub and quickly wrap them in a clean, dry towel. Gently pat them dry.
- **Dress and cuddle:** Dress your baby in clean, dry clothes, and enjoy some cuddle time. To keep your infant warm after the bath, make sure the room is comfortably heated.

Remember, a baby's skin is delicate, so use mild, baby-specific products and handle your baby gently during diaper changes and baths. You will get more confident and efficient at performing these activities with time, and it will become a natural part of your daily routine as a parent.

16.7: Baby's Sleep Time

Providing a safe and comfortable sleep environment for your baby is crucial for their health and ensuring they get adequate rest. Here is a discussion on various aspects of baby's sleep time, including crib safety, temperature, and synchronizing sleep schedules.

Crib Safety

- **Crib choice:** Start by choosing a sturdy, well-constructed crib that adheres to current safety standards. To ensure conformity, look for certificates such as Juvenile Products Manufacturers Association (JPMA).
- **Crib placement:** Do not place the crib close to windows, cords, curtains, and other potential hazards. Make sure there is only a fitted sheet in the crib, and avoid using crib bumpers, pillows, or stuffed animals, as they can pose suffocation risks. Protect your baby from direct sunlight and drafts.
- **Mattress:** Use a crib mattress that is firm and fits snugly into the crib. To avoid trapping hazards, there should be no gaps between the mattress and the crib edges.
- **Suffocation hazards:** Make sure that your baby's sleepwear does not have long strings or ties that could be a strangulation risk. Do not use loose bedding and

blankets in the crib; the better option would be to use sleep sacks or wearable blankets.

Temperature

- **Room temperature:** Maintain a suitable room temperature for your baby, ideally between 68–72°F (20–22°C).
- **Thermoregulation:** Babies are not as adept at regulating their body temperature as adults, so it is crucial to monitor them for signs of overheating or being too cold. Check their neck or back to make sure they are not very sweaty or cold. At birth, the spaces between the cranium (bones of the skull) are not completely sealed, so it is necessary to protect the head from temperature fluctuations and extremes, especially cold. A baby cap is often a good idea to mitigate this.
- **Dress appropriately:** Dress your newborn in light, breathable layers. Cotton onesies or sleepers are favorable options. Do not overdress your baby or use heavy blankets.
- **Ventilation:** Maintain proper airflow in the room to avoid overheating. If required, consider using a fan on a low setting or open a window slightly.

Synchronizing Sleep Schedules

- **Routine:** Having a regular bedtime routine helps to give your baby a sense of sleep time. This can include activities like a warm bath, gentle massage, feeding, reading a book, and dimming the lights.

- **Recognize sleep cues:** Pay attention to your baby's behavior; gestures like yawning, rubbing their eyes, or becoming fussy are possible indications that they are tired and it is time for a nap or bedtime.
- **Adjust sleep times:** Your baby's sleep patterns will change as they grow. Newborns sleep a lot and wake up frequently due to hunger, but as they get older, their sleep patterns will become more predictable. Adjust and adapt your schedule to meet the changing requirements of your infant.

Rooming-In: A Scientific Perspective

- **Bonding and attachment:** Rooming-in, or sleeping in the same room as the mother, is widely thought to be beneficial for developing early bonding and attachment between the mother and baby. This closeness can aid in promoting emotional security and the start of breastfeeding (Crenshaw, 2007).
- **Breastfeeding support:** Rooming-in allows for more frequent and convenient nursing, which has been associated with a variety of health benefits for the baby, including a lower risk of infection and enhanced nutritional intake through breast milk.
- **Temperature regulation:** The mother's proximity enables better monitoring and adjusting of the baby's temperature, particularly during the crucial early days.

- **Enhanced awareness:** The mother is able to respond to the baby's signs and wants more quickly, leading to a better understanding of the baby's behavior and overall well-being.
- **Sleep patterns:** While rooming-in may cause an initial disturbance in the mother's sleep patterns, it may eventually lead to more synchronized sleep schedules as both mother and baby adjust to each other's rhythms.
- **Overall benefits:** Rooming-in is generally looked upon as a positive practice for encouraging maternal-infant bonding, breastfeeding success, and early infant care (Theo & Drake, 2017), but individual preferences and circumstances must be considered, as some mothers may benefit from short periods of separation for rest and recuperation.

Prioritizing your baby's safety and comfort while also establishing a sleep routine that works for your family is essential. If you are concerned about your baby's sleep or safety, consult with a pediatrician or a certified sleep consultant for personalized guidance.

16.8: Scheduling Circumcision

A baby's circumcision is a medical procedure that should be discussed with a healthcare provider and is usually performed by either of the following: a pediatrician, a pediatric urologist, or an obstetrician. If you are contemplating circumcising your baby, here are some general measures to consider:

- **Consult with a healthcare professional:** Start by talking to your pediatrician, pediatric urologist, or obstetrician about the circumcision procedure. They can advise you about the procedure's benefits, risks, and the best time to have it done.
- **Timing:** Circumcision is normally performed within the first few days to weeks of a baby's life, but it can also be performed at a later age if desired. Several factors, including the baby's health and any cultural or religious considerations, can influence the date.
- **Informed consent:** Parents have to give informed consent for the procedure. To help you make an informed decision, your healthcare professional should thoroughly explain the procedure, including its risks and benefits (NHS, 2022c).
- **Select a healthcare provider:** If you decide to proceed with circumcision, find a healthcare professional who has performed the operation before. They will arrange the procedure and advise you on how to prepare your baby.
- **Preparation:** Your healthcare professional will provide you with precise instructions for preparing your baby for the circumcision procedure. This may entail not feeding for a period of time prior to surgery.
- **Procedure:** On the day of the circumcision, you will bring your baby to the healthcare center. The procedure is normally performed under local anesthesia and takes only a few minutes to complete.
- **Aftercare:** Following the circumcision, your healthcare provider will instruct you on how to care

for the surgical site as it heals. This normally involves keeping the area clean and applying antibiotic ointment as recommended.

- **Follow-up:** Schedule a follow-up appointment with your healthcare provider to confirm that the circumcision site is healing properly and that no issues have arisen.

It is worth mentioning that the decision to circumcise a baby is a personal one and may be influenced by cultural, religious, or medical factors. To make the best decision for your child's health and well-being, it is important to have open and informed discussions with your healthcare professional. Furthermore, circumcision availability and regulations may differ by country and region; therefore, it is critical to be aware of local guidelines and customs.

16.9: Obtaining Your Baby's Social Security Card

Obtaining your baby's Social Security card is needed to ensure their financial security and identity. A Social Security number (SSN) is a unique identifier that will be used for a variety of purposes throughout your child's life, such as opening a bank account, applying for government benefits, and filing taxes. Here are some guidelines on how to obtain your baby's Social Security card.

Prepare the Necessary Documents

Proof of the baby's identity, citizenship, and your personal identity as the parent or guardian will be required. Your child's birth certificate, hospital record of birth, and your photo ID (e.g., driver's license, passport) are the usual documents.

Complete the Application

To apply for a Social Security card for your infant, you must complete Form SS-5: Application for a Social Security card. You can get this form at the Social Security Administration's (SSA) website or from a local SSA office.

Select the Application Method

There are two options for submitting the application:

1. **In-person:** You can submit your application and documentation in person at your local Social Security office. To save time, make a call ahead and schedule an appointment.
2. **By mail:** You can also mail the completed application and supporting documentation to your local SSA office. Include copies of the necessary documents as well as any requested information.

Provide Proof of Citizenship

If your child was born in the United States, you must produce a copy of their birth certificate or hospital record. If your child is not a citizen of the United States, you must show proof of their immigration status, such as a Certificate of Naturalization or a Permanent Resident Card (Green Card).

Verify Parental Identity

You will be required to establish your identity as the parent or guardian. This usually requires presenting a legitimate government-issued photo ID, such as a driver's license or passport.

Submit the Application

Whether you apply in person or by mail, make sure to include the necessary documents as well as the completed Form SS-5. Ensure that all the provided information is accurate and updated.

Wait for Processing

The time it takes to process a baby's Social Security card varies, but it usually takes a few weeks. You may receive the card sooner if you file the application in person.

Receive the Social Security Card

Once the application is processed, the baby's Social Security card will be mailed to the address listed on the application form.

Safeguard the Card

Ensure your baby's eligibility for government benefits by safely keeping their Social Security card, revealing the SSN only when absolutely necessary to prevent identity misuse.

As new parents bond with their baby, being aware of emotional challenges is crucial. Differentiating between common "baby blues" and more serious conditions like post-partum depression is important. The next chapter explores these distinctions, offering valuable insights for both parents and their children in the early stages of parenthood.

Chapter 17

Depression Versus "Baby Blues" Versus Psychosis

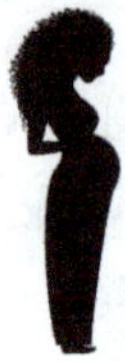

Depression is a common, long-lasting mental health condition characterized by persistent sadness and a loss of interest in activities. By contrast, "baby blues" is a temporary and milder emotional state experienced by new mothers, while postpartum psychosis is a severe mental health emergency involving hallucinations, delusions, and disorientation that requires prompt medical intervention. Here are the details of all three conditions.

17.1: Postpartum "Baby Blues"

Postpartum "baby blues" are commonly and temporarily experienced by many new mothers shortly after giving birth. This emotional state often manifests within a few days to a few weeks following childbirth and is characterized by various mild to moderate emotional symptoms. Here are some key aspects of postpartum "baby blues":

- **Common occurrence:** Baby blues are very common, affecting up to 70–80% of new mothers (American Pregnancy Association, n.d.-a). Nearly every mother experiences some degree of emotional turmoil in the days or weeks following childbirth.
- **Symptoms:** Mood swings, tearfulness, impatience, anxiety, and feelings of melancholy or overwhelm are common signs of baby blues. These feelings can be intense, but they are usually fleeting and self-limiting.
- **Duration:** Baby blues often peak between the third and fifth day after delivery and resolve on their own within two weeks. If your symptoms persist or worsen, it could be a sign of a more serious disorder like postpartum depression.
- **Causes:** The exact cause of baby blues is not known, but it is thought to be linked with the considerable hormonal changes taking place throughout pregnancy and the postpartum period. In fact, recent research findings suggest that the dramatic drop in progesterone levels after giving birth may be a significant contributor to both postpartum blues and postpartum depression (Trifu et al., 2019). Sleep deprivation, physical discomfort, and the transition to new motherhood can also contribute to these emotional changes.
- **Support:** It is essential for mothers experiencing baby blues to be in a supportive and understanding setting. Partners, family members, and friends can all help by providing emotional support, assisting with domestic duties, and ensuring the new mother gets enough rest.

- **Self-care:** Engaging in self-care routines can potentially alleviate baby blues symptoms. This may entail getting enough rest when the baby naps, eating a well-balanced diet, doing some light exercise when possible, and seeking out moments of mindful relaxation.
- **Communication:** It is necessary to maintain open and honest communication with healthcare providers. Women should not be afraid to talk to their obstetrician, midwife, or primary care physician about their emotional condition, as they can offer advice and check for warning signs of more serious postpartum mood disorders.

17.2: Postpartum Depression

Postpartum depression (PPD) is a mental health disorder that affects some women shortly after giving birth. A mother can experience melancholy, hopelessness, and anguish that go beyond the ordinary "baby blues" experienced by many new mothers. While baby blues are usually mild and short-lived, PPD is more severe and can have a substantial effect on a mother's ability to function and care for herself and her baby. Here is a more in-depth look at postpartum depression.

- **Timing:** PPD usually begins within the first few weeks following childbirth; however, it may develop at any moment during the first year postpartum.
- **Symptoms:** PPD symptoms vary in severity and may include

- **Persistent sadness:** A profound and lasting sadness that does not improve with time.
- **Loss of interest or pleasure:** A loss of interest in previously enjoyable activities.
- **Fatigue and lack of energy:** Constant fatigue and inability to regain energy despite rest.
- **Changes in appetite or weight:** Significant changes in eating habits that may result in weight gain or loss.
- **Sleep disturbances:** Difficulty falling or staying asleep, even when the baby is asleep.
- **Feelings of guilt or worthlessness:** Believing you're a bad mother or incapable of caring for your child.
- **Difficulty concentrating:** Having difficulty focusing or making decisions.

In some severe instances, mothers may have troubling thoughts about hurting themselves or their baby, but it's highly unlikely that they would act on these thoughts.

- **Causes:** What exactly causes PPD is not fully understood, but it is possibly due to a combination of physical, emotional, and social factors (Pietrangelo, 2022). Hormonal changes, such as a sudden drop in estrogen and progesterone levels after childbirth, can be involved. A personal or family history of depression, high levels of stress, a pre-existing deficiency of the mood-regulating hormone serotonin, a lack of social support, and adverse living situations can also be risk factors.

- **Impact:** PPD can have serious effects on both the mother and her child. A mother suffering from PPD may find it difficult to bond with her newborn, which can have an impact on the child's emotional development. Furthermore, the mother's physical health may suffer as a result of inadequate sleep, poor nutrition, and a lack of self-care.
- **Treatment:** PPD is treatable and early intervention is crucial. Treatment options may include
- **Therapy:** Effective forms of therapy can be individual or group therapy, such as cognitive-behavioral therapy (CBT) or interpersonal therapy (IPT).
- **Medication:** Some cases may require the use of antidepressant medications, particularly for moderate to severe PPD.
- **Support groups:** Joining a PPD moms' support group can offer emotional support and create a sense of belonging in a caring community.
- **Self-care:** Practicing self-care, like getting enough sleep, eating healthy food, and engaging in physical activity, is necessary.
- **Social support:** Family and friends can be invaluable in providing practical and emotional support for the mother.

It is important to realize that PPD is a medical condition, not a weakness or an indication of inadequate mothering skills. Seeking help and support is crucial for both the mother's well-being and the baby's healthy development.

17.3: Postpartum Psychosis

Postpartum psychosis is classified as a psychiatric emergency due to the sudden development of symptoms that can be extremely disruptive and even life-threatening. Here's an in-depth look at postpartum psychosis:

Onset and Timing

Postpartum psychosis usually appears within the first two weeks of childbirth, but it can happen as late as the first few months.

Symptoms

- **Delusions:** Women with postpartum psychosis usually have delusions, which are firmly held false beliefs. These delusions may be about the baby, such as feeling the baby is possessed, needing to protect the baby from harm, or that they have a special mission related to the baby.
- **Hallucinations:** Hallucinations are common in postpartum psychosis, particularly auditory hallucinations (hearing voices).
- **Mood disturbances:** There are also severe mood swings such as extreme agitation, exhilaration, or severe depression.
- **Disorganized thoughts and behavior:** Disorganized thinking and behavior are distinguishing features. Other signs include confusion, fast-talking, impulsivity, or erratic behavior.

- **Lack of insight:** Often, women suffering from postpartum psychosis are unaware that they are suffering from a mental disease, which is referred to as a lack of insight.
- **Paranoia:** Another potential indication is paranoia or intense distrust or suspicion of others.

Risk Factors

While the actual cause of postpartum psychosis is unknown, it is thought to be a combination of biological, hormonal, and psychological factors. A history of bipolar disorder, a previous episode of postpartum psychosis, a family history of mood disorders, or a recent stressful life event are all risk factors (NHS, 2020b).

Diagnosis

Diagnosis is primarily clinical and based on the presence of specific symptoms. Physical and laboratory tests may also be performed by healthcare practitioners to rule out any underlying medical disorders that could mirror the symptoms.

Treatment

- Postpartum psychosis is a medical emergency that requires immediate intervention to safeguard both the mother and the infant. Usually, hospitalization is required.
- Treatment may include a combination of medication and psychotherapy. Antipsychotic medications are often prescribed to treat psychotic symptoms, and

mood stabilizers or antidepressants may be considered if a mood disorder is present.

- Psychotherapy, such as cognitive-behavioral therapy (CBT) or supportive therapy, can help the mother cope with her experiences and develop strategies for managing her symptoms.

Prognosis

- Postpartum psychosis has a relatively favorable prognosis when treated promptly and appropriately. Many women heal completely and have no recurrence of problems.
- However, if not treated, postpartum psychosis can have serious repercussions, such as self-harm or harm to the baby.

Impact on Mother and Family

- Postpartum psychosis is a traumatic experience for both the affected mother and her family. Support from loved ones and healthcare professionals is vital during the healing process.
- Family members should be informed about the condition and encouraged to seek help if they suspect a loved one is suffering from postpartum psychosis.

17.4: How to Recognize When to Seek Help for Postpartum Emotions

Recognizing when to seek help for postpartum emotions is critical for both the mother's and the baby's well-being. Here are some key signs and suggestions to help you realize when it is time to seek postpartum emotional support:

- **Persistent and severe mood swings:** Due to hormonal fluctuations, it is normal to experience mood swings after giving birth. However, if these mood swings continue and get more intense, it could be an indication of a more serious problem.
- **Feeling overwhelmed:** Feeling overwhelmed, apprehensive, or always worried about the baby's well-being to the extent that it interferes with your routine life is a red flag.
- **Extreme fatigue:** While fatigue is a normal occurrence with a newborn, extreme exhaustion that does not ease with rest or sleep may indicate a problem.
- **Loss of interest or pleasure:** If you no longer enjoy activities or interests that you once did, this could be an indication of depression.
- **Changes in appetite or weight:** Significant changes in eating habits or noticeable weight gain/loss may be signs of a mood disorder.
- **Difficulty bonding with the baby:** Struggling to form a strong bond with or nurture your infant, despite your sincere desire to do so, may be a sign of postpartum depression or anxiety.

- **Intense irritability or anger:** Frequent outbursts of anger or irritability that are not normal behavior for you may be a sign of a mood disorder.
- **Thinking about hurting yourself or the baby:** It is crucial not to disregard any thoughts related to self-harm or harming the baby.
- **Social withdrawal:** Avoiding social engagements or distancing yourself from friends and family can be an indication that something is awry.
- **Sleep disturbances:** Significant changes in your sleep routine, like insomnia or excessive sleep, may signal a possible mood disorder.
- **Physical symptoms:** Postpartum mood disorders are occasionally accompanied by unexplained physical symptoms like migraines, stomachaches, or chest pain.
- **Difficulty concentrating:** An inability to focus or concentrate on tasks, no matter how trivial, can indicate a mood disorder.

If you or someone you know is experiencing some of these symptoms and they are persistent (lasting for more than a couple of weeks) and interfering with everyday functioning, it is critical that you seek professional care as soon as possible. The following are the measures to take:

- **Talk to a healthcare provider:** Begin by talking to your obstetrician, primary care physician, or a mental health expert about your feelings and symptoms. They can provide a preliminary assessment and recommend appropriate treatment options.

- **Therapy:** This has proven to be useful in treating postpartum mood problems, particularly cognitive-behavioral therapy (CBT) and interpersonal therapy.
- **Medication:** In some cases, medication, such as antidepressants, may be administered to help stabilize mood and manage symptoms. This is often used along with therapy.
- **Involve a support system:** Ask friends and family for help with childcare, housework, and emotional support. Don't hesitate to ask for help when needed.
- **Self-care:** Prioritize self-care activities such as exercise, healthy eating, and enough sleep. These can have a substantial impact on mood improvement.

Bear in mind that reaching out for help is a sign of strength, not weakness. Early intervention can lead to a faster recovery and a happier postpartum experience for both the mother and the baby.

17.5: Is It Possible for My Spouse/Partner to Experience Postpartum Depression?

Yes, a spouse or partner can suffer from depression or a mood disorder after the birth of a child. However, this may not be termed "postpartum depression" in the strictest clinical sense. The term "postpartum depression" is commonly used to describe the mood disorder that affects some mothers after childbirth, but it is important to recognize that other members of the family, such as fathers, partners, and even adoptive parents, may also experience significant emotional and psychological difficulties during this time.

When examining the probability of a spouse or partner experiencing postpartum depression or a related mood disorder, take into account the following factors:

- **Paternal postpartum depression:** Dads are also known to experience emotions like depression and anxiety after welcoming their baby. This is often referred to as paternal postpartum depression. The signs are quite similar to what mothers experience with postpartum depression, including feelings of sadness, irritability, fatigue, shifts in sleep and eating patterns, and difficulty forming a strong connection with their baby (Horsager-Boehrer, 2021).
- **Contributing factors:** Several factors can cause a spouse or partner to experience depression during the postpartum period. These can be hormonal changes, inadequate sleep, higher stress levels, changes in family relationships, financial pressures, and feelings of inadequacy as a parent or partner.
- **Impact on the family:** When a spouse or partner suffers from postpartum depression, the entire family suffers. It may strain the relationship, impair parenting quality, and have long-term ramifications for the child's development.
- **Seeking help:** It is essential for both partners to recognize the symptoms of postpartum depression or other mood disorders and to reach out for help when needed. Talking to a healthcare provider, therapist, or counselor can help with this. Therapy, medication, support groups, and changes in lifestyle are all possible treatment options.

- **Support and communication:** Open and caring interaction is essential for both couples throughout this trying time. Sharing feelings, getting support from friends and family, and working together to handle stress and responsibilities can all help in improving the situation.
- **Prevention:** It can be beneficial to take steps to prevent postpartum depression in either partner. This can include emotional and practical preparation for a child's arrival, seeking prenatal education and counseling, and establishing a strong support network.

As we conclude our discussion on postpartum emotional issues, it is important to realize that fathers and partners can also suffer from comparable mood disorders during this period. Seeking help and treatment when needed is crucial for the well-being of both the individual and the family. Now, move on to the practical and physical aspects of postpartum life in the next chapter, where you will learn how to care for and manage the changes your body undergoes throughout this transformative journey.

Chapter 18

Managing Your Postpartum Body

During the postpartum period, a woman's body experiences numerous changes and challenges, some of which are unexpected and even distressing. This chapter explores various aspects of postpartum body management, addressing concerns ranging from physical changes like breast enlargement and potential complications like clogged milk ducts and mastitis to the sensitive subject of resuming sexual activity following childbirth.

18.1: Breast Enlargement With Milk (Engorgement and Leaking)

Breast enlargement with milk, also known as engorgement, is a common postpartum experience for new mothers. This occurs when the breast tissue fills with milk, causing the breasts to swell, become uncomfortable, and sometimes painful. Engorgement usually starts a few days after childbirth, when a mother's milk supply increases to fulfill the demands of her baby. Here's a more detailed explanation of this aspect of postpartum body management.

Engorgement

This is a painful condition that can leave the breasts feeling hard and swollen. As the mammary glands fill up with milk, blood flow to the breast tissue increases. Engorgement needs to be properly managed by new mothers to avoid more discomfort and complications.

- **Relief techniques:** Warm compresses or warm showers before nursing or pumping might help relieve engorgement. Cold packs applied between feedings can help minimize swelling and soreness. To successfully drain the breasts, it is necessary that the baby latches properly during nursing.
- **Pumping:** In cases where breastfeeding becomes difficult, using a breast pump can help empty the breasts and give relief. However, it is imperative to avoid over-pumping, as this can signal the body to produce even more milk, worsening the issue.

Leaking

This is another common occurrence related to breast enlargement. This happens when surplus milk drips or sprays from the breasts, usually when a mother is neither nursing or pumping. Leaking can be unpredictable and sometimes embarrassing, but it is a normal aspect of the postpartum period.

- **Breast pads:** Many women use breast pads to manage leaking, which can be inserted inside a bra to absorb any milk leakage. Disposable and reusable options are available to cater to individual preferences.
- **Breastfeeding bras:** Purchasing comfortable and supportive nursing bras can assist in providing better support for engorged breasts and can also accommodate breast pads.

It should be understood that breast enlargement, engorgement, and leaking are usually temporary issues that resolve as the body adjusts to the baby's feeding patterns. However, if engorgement becomes severe or persistent, or if there are signs of mastitis (which will be discussed later), it is important to seek counsel and support from a healthcare provider or a lactation consultant. Managing breast changes is a vital aspect of postpartum care, and with proper strategies, most moms can successfully navigate this phase while supplying their infant with essential nourishment.

18.2: Clogged Milk Ducts

Clogged milk ducts, or plugged milk ducts, can be a common concern for breastfeeding mothers. They occur when one of the breast's milk ducts becomes plugged, restricting the flow of milk.

Causes

- Clogged milk ducts can result from a variety of factors, such as inadequate milk removal from the breast during breastfeeding.
- Pressure on the breast, due to wearing a tight-fitting bra, can contribute to duct blockages.
- A duct might also become blocked as a result of an abrupt change in the baby's feeding habit or position.

Symptoms

- A painful lump or knot in the breast is the most prevalent symptom.
- The affected area may seem red and feel warm to the touch.
- While breastfeeding, some moms may experience discomfort or pain from the affected breast.
- Milk flow from the affected breast may decrease, causing concerns about milk supply.

Treatment and Prevention

- To alleviate a clogged milk duct, applying warm compresses to the affected area before breastfeeding can assist in relaxing the duct and improving milk flow.
- Gently massaging the breast while breastfeeding, focusing on the area with the blockage, can encourage the milk to flow.

- It is possible to avoid future blockages by ensuring proper positioning and latching during breastfeeding.
- Changing feeding positions or using breast compression techniques during feeds may aid in the prevention of recurrent duct blockages.
- Consult a healthcare physician if the blockage persists or is linked with infection symptoms (such as fever), as this may necessitate medical treatment.

Impact on Breastfeeding

- Clogged milk ducts can obstruct milk flow, potentially resulting in reduced milk supply.
- If they are not treated promptly, they can progress to a more serious illness known as mastitis, which is a painful breast infection.
- Timely management is imperative to sustaining breastfeeding and avoiding complications.

In general, clogged milk ducts are a common problem for breastfeeding mothers, but they are usually treatable with home remedies and breastfeeding practices. However, it is essential to seek medical help if the symptoms persist or intensify in order to protect both the mother's and the baby's health.

18.3: Mastitis (Inflammation of Blocked Ducts)

Mastitis is a condition that can affect breastfeeding women and is caused by inflammation of the milk ducts. This painful ailment develops when breast milk does not flow freely, resulting in infection and discomfort. Here's a closer look at mastitis:

- **Causes:** Mastitis can result from a combination of factors, such as milk duct blockages, milk accumulation, and bacterial infection. Sometimes, it can be caused by poor breastfeeding positioning or latch issues.
- **Symptoms:** These commonly include a hot, swollen, and painful breast, often accompanied by a fever or chills. The affected breast may become red and painful to touch (NHS Choices, 2023).
- **Treatment:** Mastitis is often treated with a combination of methods. Regular breastfeeding or pumping on the affected breast can help clear the blockage. Applying warm compresses before breastfeeding can also help alleviate discomfort. In certain cases, antibiotics may be recommended to cure any underlying infection.
- **Prevention:** Using proper nursing practices and maintaining breast hygiene can help avoid mastitis. Ensuring that your baby latches correctly and fully drains the breasts during feeds can lower the chance of milk duct blockages.
- **Consulting a healthcare provider:** If you suspect you have mastitis or if your symptoms worsen despite home treatments, you should see a healthcare practitioner at once. They can provide a clear diagnosis and suggest appropriate treatment.

Mastitis can be a difficult and painful experience for new mothers, but it can be effectively controlled with immediate treatment and proper care, allowing breastfeeding to proceed uninterrupted.

18.4: Sex After Childbirth

For many new mothers, sexual activity after childbirth can be a complicated and sensitive subject. Here are a few pointers worth noting.

Pain Concerns

It is very common to feel some discomfort or even pain during intercourse following childbirth, especially in the initial weeks. This discomfort can be the result of physical changes, healing processes, or hormonal changes. It is essential to be open with your partner about any discomfort or pain you may be experiencing and consider taking things slowly to enable your body to recuperate.

When It's Okay to Resume Sex

The timeline for resuming sexual activity can be different for every woman. Generally, healthcare professionals recommend waiting until any vaginal bleeding or discharge has ended, any tears or episiotomies have healed, and you are physically comfortable. This might span from a few weeks to several months. It is advisable to consult with your healthcare provider for personalized guidance, depending on your specific situation.

Necessary Precautions

Using a water-based lubricant can help lessen friction and discomfort during intercourse. It is also crucial to practice safe sex and use contraception unless you are all set and ready for another pregnancy. Additionally, maintaining proper pelvic floor muscle strength by performing exercises like Kegels can improve sex comfort.

Lack of Desire

Due to hormonal changes, weariness, stress, and the duties of caring for a newborn, many women feel a drop in sexual desire after childbirth (Gutzeit et al., 2020). It is essential to understand that this is normal and does not indicate a lack of love or attraction for your partner. Discuss your feelings with your partner freely, and consider receiving help from a therapist or counselor if necessary.

Benefits Versus Risks

While resuming sexual activity might help you retain intimacy and connection with your spouse, you must prioritize your physical and emotional well-being. Sexual activity before your body is ready may cause discomfort or difficulties. Weigh the benefits of intimacy against possible risks, and always put your comfort and health first.

When to Resume Contraception

If you are not ready for another pregnancy, talk to your doctor about contraception options before resuming sexual activity. Barrier techniques such as condoms and nonhormonal methods such as copper IUDs may be appropriate for many postpartum women; however, hormonal options should also be considered.

Remember that every woman's postpartum experience is unique, so there is no rush to return to sexual activity. Open communication with your partner and seeking advice from a healthcare expert can assist you in maintaining your physical and mental well-being throughout this transition period. Don't forget to prioritize regular postnatal check-ups for both you and your newborn—they provide guidance and reassurance as you move on to the next chapter of your postpartum journey.

Chapter 19

Postnatal Check-Up for Mom and Baby

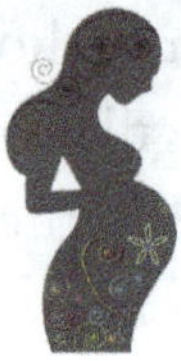

Following the joyous arrival of a new baby, it is essential that both mother and infant are properly cared for during the postnatal period. This crucial phase involves scheduled check-ups to monitor the health and well-being of both mom and baby, answering questions about when to expect these check-ups, whether they will take place before or after leaving the hospital, what happens during these visits, and what essentials to bring along for a full evaluation of postpartum health.

19.1: How Soon After Birth Should I Expect a Post-Birth Check-Up?

The timing of a post-birth check-up is crucial for safeguarding both mother and baby's well-being. Here is what to expect:

- **Within the first week:** It is generally recommended that both the mother and the baby receive their initial postnatal check-ups within the first week of birth.

This enables medical professionals to closely monitor the early stages of recuperation and development.

- **First 24 to 48 hours:** In certain cases, the infant may have their first check-up within the first 24 to 48 hours of birth, while the mother may have her initial examination while still in the hospital.
- **Hospital discharge:** If you had a hospital delivery, your baby will normally receive their first check-up before being discharged. Staff at the hospital will make certain that the infant is stable, feeds well, and has no immediate health concerns.
- **Mother's check-up:** For moms, the time of the post-birth check-up may vary. Some healthcare practitioners prefer to conduct an initial assessment before discharge, while others prefer to schedule a follow-up visit within a week.
- **Home births:** If you have a home birth, your midwife or healthcare provider will usually visit you and the baby within the first few days to confirm that you and the baby are both healthy and recuperating well.
- **Preterm or complicated births:** Postnatal check-ups may be more regular and immediate to treat any potential health issues.
- **Follow-up schedule:** Following the initial post-birth check-up, your healthcare practitioner will discuss a follow-up schedule that caters to your unique needs. This schedule may include additional visits during the first six weeks after delivery.
- **Telehealth options:** In some cases, especially if you and your baby are in good health, telehealth visits for

specific postnatal check-ups may be a possibility, allowing you to receive care from the comfort of your own home.

Be sure to consult with your healthcare provider or pediatrician regarding the exact timing of post-birth check-ups, as this can differ depending on individual circumstances and the health of both mother and baby. These check-ups are very important in paving the way for a healthy start for both you and your newborn.

19.2: Is My Postnatal Check-up Scheduled Before or After I Leave the Hospital?

The scheduling of your postnatal check-up depends on a number of factors, including hospital policy, your medical history, and the health of both you and your baby. Here's a closer look at when your postnatal check-up should take place in relation to your hospital stay:

- **In-hospital check-ups:** Many hospitals perform initial postnatal check-ups while you're still in the hospital. These in-hospital visits are most common within the first 24 to 48 hours following delivery. This time is used by healthcare providers to assess the immediate well-being of both you and your newborn.
- **Transition to home:** Following the initial in-hospital assessment, you will be discharged to go home. The time of this discharge can vary, with shorter stays for uncomplicated births and longer stays for difficult births.

- **Post-discharge check-ups:** Regardless of when you leave the hospital, post-discharge check-ups are part of your postnatal care. These appointments are usually made within a week or two of leaving the hospital.
- **Special circumstances:** If you or your baby have medical concerns or complications that require monitoring, your healthcare provider may schedule additional check-ups before or after you are discharged from the hospital.
- **Home visits:** In situations like home births, postnatal check-ups may be done at home by your chosen healthcare professional, including a midwife.

Put simply, the scheduling of your postnatal check-up can include both in-hospital assessments shortly after birth and post-discharge appointments within the first few weeks following birth. The specific schedule will be determined by your specific circumstances and the recommendations of your healthcare provider. It is vital to maintain contact with your healthcare team to properly understand your postnatal care plan and receive the necessary support during this critical period.

19.3: Expectations at the Postpartum Check-up Visit

New moms should expect a full assessment of their health and well-being, as well as a review of their newborn's growth and development, during their postpartum check-up visit. Here are some key expectations for this important visit:

Physical Examination

- Your healthcare practitioner will perform a comprehensive physical examination to examine your postpartum recovery, including the healing of any incisions or stitches.
- Blood pressure, heart rate, and temperature will be checked to verify they are within normal ranges.
- Breast health will be assessed for any signs of disorders such as engorgement or mastitis.

Emotional Well-Being

Your mental and emotional well-being will be addressed. It's a chance to disclose your feelings of postpartum depression or anxiety so that your physician can provide support and direction.

Birth Control Options

The consultation will include a discussion of birth control alternatives to assist you in selecting a method that meets your family planning goals.

Breastfeeding Support

If you're nursing, your healthcare practitioner can provide advice and address any concerns you have about your baby's latch, milk supply, or other breastfeeding-related issues.

Infant Development

Weight gain, height, and head circumference measurements will be taken to assess your baby's growth and development. Developmental milestones will be discussed as well.

Vaccinations

During the visit, your healthcare practitioner will discuss your baby's vaccination schedule and administer any necessary vaccines.

Postpartum Recovery

You'll get the chance to talk about any discomfort or pain you're still feeling after childbirth, as well as any remaining symptoms or concerns.

Birth Control

If you are sexually active and do not intend to have another pregnancy soon, birth control options will be explored and a plan will be decided upon.

Nutrition and Exercise

To help you recover your strength and energy, your provider may advise you on postpartum diet and safe exercise methods.

Questions and Concerns

This is a perfect opportunity to ask questions or raise worries regarding your postpartum experience, your baby's health, or any other related issues.

Future Care Plan

To ensure that both you and your baby receive appropriate follow-up treatment, a plan will be drawn up for future healthcare visits and check-ups.

19.4: What Do I Need to Take With Me?

When preparing for your postnatal check-up, make sure you have everything you need for a full assessment of your post-partum health. Here's a list of items to consider bringing with you:

- **Medical records and ID:** Bring any medical records pertaining to your pregnancy, labor, and delivery. This comprises your prenatal care records, hospital discharge summary, and identification (driver's license, insurance cards, or hospital ID). Bringing your medical records may not be necessary if you will continue seeing the same OB/GYN you saw for your prenatal care. Furthermore, most hospital systems are able to transmit health records electronically to one another once the patient signs a release.
- **Prescription medications:** Bring any medications that you were taking during your pregnancy or after giving birth. This allows your doctor to assess your medication regimen and make any necessary changes.
- **List of questions:** Make a list of any questions or concerns you have about your postpartum recovery, newborn care, breastfeeding, or any emotional difficulties you're experiencing. This guarantees that

essential topics are not forgotten during your appointment.

- **Baby essentials:** If your postnatal check-up includes an examination of your newborn, bring diapers, wipes, a blanket, and a change of clothes. Furthermore, if you are breastfeeding, you might want to bring items such as a nursing cover or a breast pump.
- **Breastfeeding log:** If you're breastfeeding, maintain a record of your baby's feeding habits, including feeding times and duration. This might be useful when discussing any worries or issues with your healthcare provider.
- **Support person:** Bringing a support person, such as your partner or a trusted family member or friend, is generally a good idea. During the appointment, they can offer emotional support, help with the baby, and take notes.
- **Comfort items:** Postpartum check-ups can be physically and emotionally stressful, so bring items that provide comfort, like a water bottle, snacks, or a cozy sweater.
- **Insurance information:** Make sure you have easy access to your insurance information, including your insurance card and any required authorization forms. This will help to streamline your appointment's billing procedure.

You can make the most of your postnatal check-up by being well-prepared and organized, addressing any concerns, and obtaining the guidance and support you require for a healthy and seamless postpartum recovery.

Chapter 20

Bonus Chapter—Healthy Recipes to Crave!

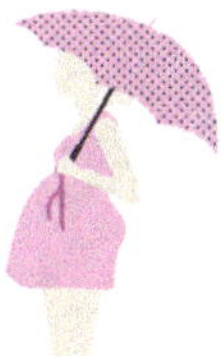

Sample First-Trimester Recipes

Breakfast/Brunch Recipe: Banana Berry Pancakes (for Morning Sickness)

Ingredients

- 2 organic eggs
- 1/4 tsp gluten-free baking powder
- 1/2 tsp cinnamon
- 1 tbsp coconut flour
- 1 banana, mashed
- 1 tsp coconut oil, extra virgin
- 1/2 cup fresh or frozen mixed berries
- 1/4 cup Greek yogurt
- 1 tbsp pumpkin seeds
- 1/2 lime, zested

Instructions

1. Combine the eggs, baking powder, cinnamon, and coconut flour in a mixing bowl.
2. Add the mashed banana and, if necessary, adjust the thickness with water.
3. Cook small pancakes in coconut oil until done on both sides.
4. Top and enjoy with yogurt, berries, pumpkin seeds, and lime zest.

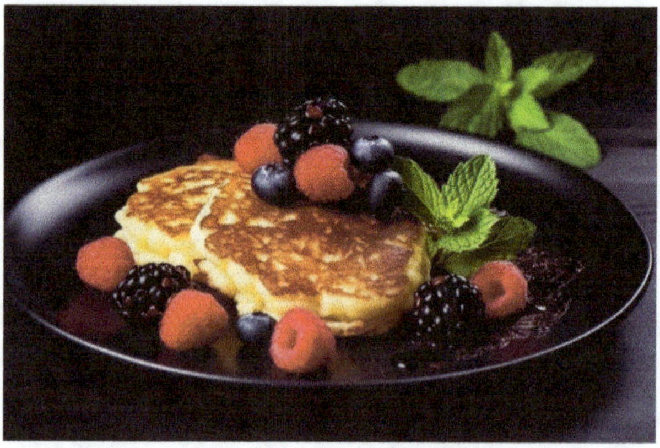

Banana Berry Pancakes

Dinner Recipe: Pesto-Stuffed Chicken with Folate-Rich Veggies

Ingredients

- 2 chicken breasts
- handful of finely chopped spinach

- crumbled feta cheese
- 2 shallots
- 2 garlic cloves
- 1 zucchini
- 1 cup of mushrooms
- 1 cup chicken stock
- pesto sauce

Instructions

1. In a mixing bowl, combine pesto, feta, and spinach.
2. Make a pouch out of each of the chicken breasts and stuff with the prepared ingredients.
3. Put the chicken in a pan and cook for 10–15 minutes over high heat, skin side down.
4. Cut shallots, garlic, zucchini, and mushrooms into slices.
5. Turn the chicken, add the stock, and cook for a further 15 minutes.
6. Remove the chicken and set aside.
7. In the same pan, add shallots, garlic, zucchini, and mushrooms, and cook for 2–3 minutes more.
8. Arrange vegetables on a plate, then top with sliced chicken. Ready to serve!

This dinner is full of nutrients, including folate from spinach and zucchini, essential for the baby's development in the first trimester.

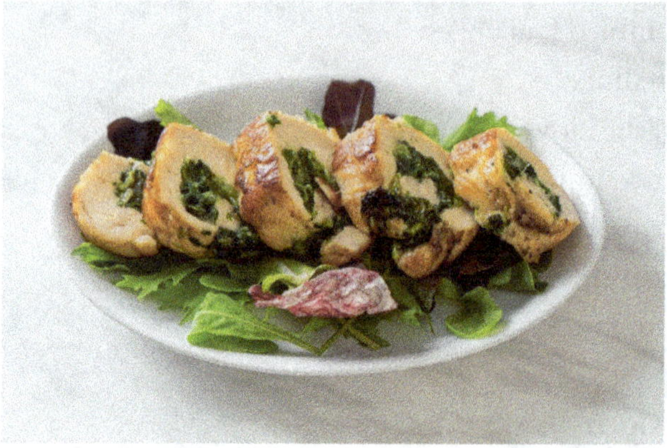

Pesto-Stuffed Chicken with Folate-Rich Veggies

Sample Second-Trimester Recipes

Breakfast/Brunch Recipe: Yogurt Crunch

Ingredients

- 1 cup rolled oats
- 1 tbsp olive oil
- 2 tbsp maple syrup
- 1/3 cup blanched almonds, chopped
- 1/3 cup chopped pecans
- 1/3 cup dried apples, chopped
- 1/3 cup dried apricots, chopped
- 1 tbsp butter
- 1/2 cup of yogurt

Instructions

1. Combine oats, olive oil, and maple syrup in a mixing bowl.

2. Spread the mixture on a greased baking tray and bake for 5 minutes.
3. Bake for a further 7 minutes after adding the almonds and pecans.
4. Place in a bowl and leave it aside to cool.
5. Mix in the dried apricots, apples, and yogurt.
6. Serve for a nutritious second-trimester breakfast/brunch!

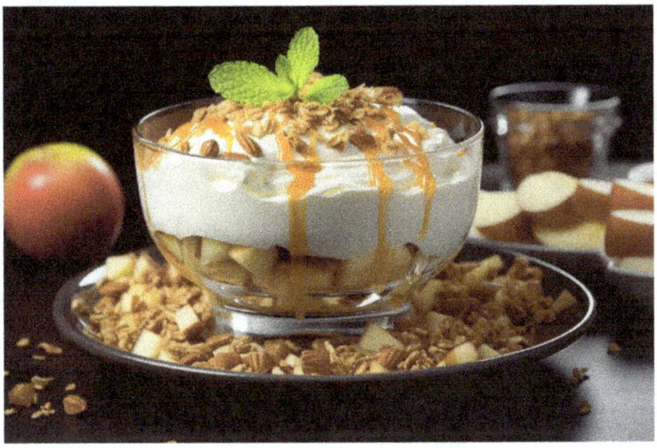

Yoghurt Crunch

Dinner Recipe: Shrimp and Pea Risotto

Ingredients

- 10 ounces of shrimp
- 1 onion, diced
- arborio rice, 2 cups
- 2 cups stock (vegetable or fish)
- 1 cup of frozen peas
- 1 can of coconut milk

- butter
- 1 tsp turmeric

Instructions

1. Cook diced onions till tender, then add 1 tsp turmeric and butter and stir.
2. Add rice.
3. Gradually stir in the stock until half of it has been absorbed, then pour in the coconut milk.
4. Continue to add stock until it is completely absorbed.
5. Add frozen peas.
6. Cook shrimp separately in butter and turmeric.
7. Mix shrimp with the risotto. Ready to serve!

This creamy and slightly spicy shrimp risotto is rich in protein, omega-3 fatty acids, and vitamins—excellent for the second trimester of pregnancy.

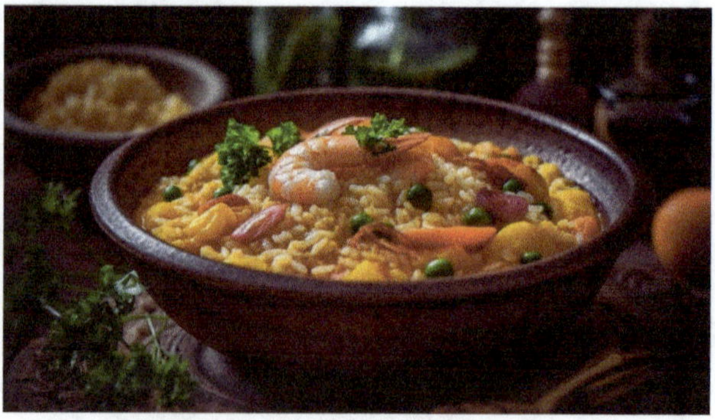

Shrimp and Pea Risotto

Sample Third-Trimester Recipes

Breakfast/Brunch Recipe: Steak and Veggie Breakfast Hash

Ingredients

- 2 tbsp of grass-fed butter
- 8 oz grass-fed steak cut into one-inch squares
- 4 ounces chopped cauliflower florets
- 1 medium-sized yellow onion, chopped
- 1/2 red bell pepper, sliced
- 1/2 yellow bell pepper, sliced
- 1/2 jalapeño pepper, finely chopped
- 1 tbsp freshly chopped parsley

Instructions

1. Heat 1 tbsp of butter in a spacious frying pan on medium-high heat.
2. Season steak chunks with salt and pepper and sear on each side until cooked to preference. To keep warm, remove from the pan and tent with foil.
3. Reduce the heat and add 1 tbsp of butter to the skillet.
4. When the butter has ceased frothing, add the cauliflower and simmer for about 2 minutes, stirring periodically. Add onions and cook until the edges of the onions begin to brown, then mix in the peppers. Enhance the flavor by adding a pinch of salt and a dash of pepper according to your taste.

5. When the peppers are crisp-tender and the vegetables are ready, add the steak cubes and any residual juices. Before serving, sprinkle with parsley.
6. Add a pinch of salt and a sprinkle of freshly ground black pepper according to your preferences.

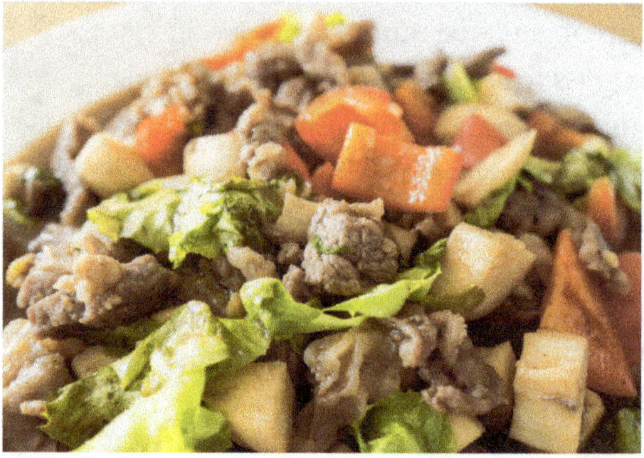

Steak and Veggie Breakfast Hash

Dinner Recipe: Thai Chicken Bake

Ingredients

- 4 chicken breasts
- 2 zucchinis
- 1 onion
- 1 red/green pepper
- 1 can of coconut milk
- 1 can diced tomatoes
- cilantro, freshly chopped
- cilantro, turmeric, and cumin

- juice from one lime
- whole-grain rice

Instructions

1. Season the chicken with the spice mixture and lime juice.
2. Place the sliced vegetables in a tray and combine with the coconut milk and tomatoes.
3. Place chicken on top and bake at 350°F for 40 minutes.
4. Serve the chicken with cooked rice after garnishing with cilantro.

This third-trimester recipe is easy—just assemble, bake, and enjoy the flavors of Thai cuisine.

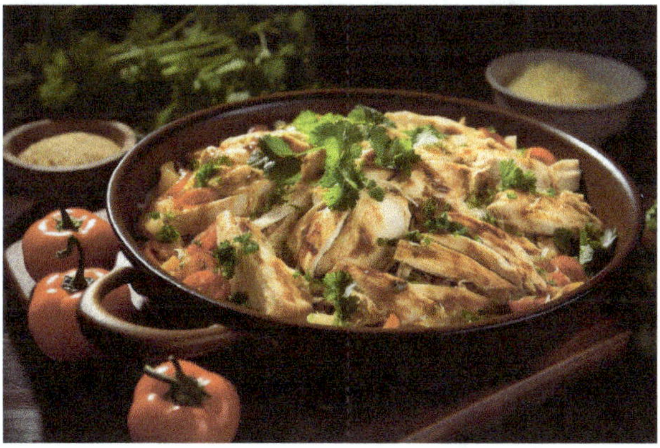

Thai Chicken Bake

These recipes cater to both the nutritional needs and occasional cravings of pregnant moms, offering a delicious and healthy culinary experience during pregnancy. So, savor each bite on this wonderful journey to motherhood!

Afterword

Now that you have reached the end of *Pregnancy, Childbirth & Your Newborn*, I hope you found this journey through the realms of pregnancy and childbirth both informative and empowering. This compact handbook has been designed to equip you with essential knowledge and practical insights as you prepare for one of life's most profound experiences: motherhood.

Throughout the pages of this book, you have walked through the intricate phases of pregnancy and childbirth. You have learned how to prepare your body for conception, navigated the rollercoaster of trimesters, understood the labor process, welcomed your baby into the world, and embarked on the "fourth trimester" of postpartum and newborn care. Additionally, the bonus chapter provided you with ideas for delightful, healthy recipes suitable for the different stages of pregnancy.

Remember that this journey has not been about just gaining information, but one of change and self-discovery. You have learned about the incredible changes your body undergoes to nurture and bring forth new life. You have had the opportunity to explore various approaches to childbirth, acquiring the necessary information to make informed decisions about your own birthing experience. You have also discovered the joys and drawbacks of early motherhood and the importance of self-care during the postpartum period.

Before you turn the final page, I would like to convey my sincere hope that this book has served as a valuable resource for you. That it has provided you with the information and guidance you needed at this pivotal stage in your life. More importantly, I hope it has offered you reassurance, encouragement, and the confidence to embark on the magnificent journey of pregnancy and motherhood.

I also encourage you to share your thoughts and experiences with others. Your feedback can serve as a guiding light for expectant mothers who will follow in your footsteps. Whether through word of mouth, online reviews, or just recommending this book to a friend, you have the power to impact the lives of those around you.

Finally, I would like to express my gratitude for entrusting *Pregnancy, Childbirth & Your Newborn* to be your companion on this remarkable journey. It has been an honor to accompany you through this transformative time in your life. Your story as a mother is just starting, and it promises to be a memorable one. As you conclude this chapter and embrace the adventure of motherhood, know that you are well-prepared, informed, and capable of dealing with the joys and challenges that await you.

Congratulations on your pregnancy, and may the days ahead be filled with love, laughter, and the endless delights that come with parenting. Thank you for choosing this book, and you have my best wishes for your exciting journey ahead.

Thank You & A Free Gift for You!

I hope you have enjoyed this pregnancy book, created to guide you through the nine months of your unique pregnancy journey. If you loved or learned from this book, kindly **leave us a review** through your Amazon purchase account. Your feedback/review means so much to small, independent authors and publishers like us. As you welcome your bundle of joy, remember that our team is available to support you and your growing family with resources that cater to every need that you may have.

Check out the author profile page of JK Karliese on your Amazon Marketplace, to preview and shop other publications by the same author and for more tips and strategies!

Scan the QR code below to leave a review ***for Pregnancy Childbirth & Your Newborn Simplified*** by JK Karliese:

SCAN ME

To show our appreciation, here's a FREE gift for you: a guide to help keep your baby safe

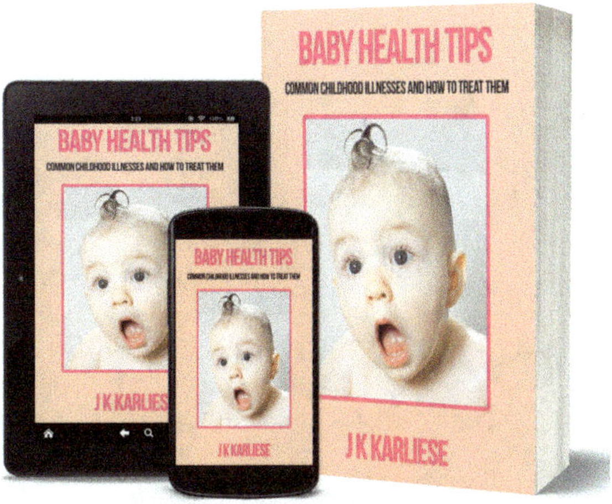

To redeem your free ebook gift, click the link below:

CLICK HERE FOR YOUR FREE EBOOK

https://subscribepage.io/Karliese-Baby-Health-Tips

References

Abdulkareem, T. A., & Eidan, S. M. (2017). *Ectopic pregnancy: diagnosis, prevention and management.* IntechOpen. https://www.intechopen.-com/chapters/57672

ACOG. (2020a, May). *How to tell when labor begins.* ACOG. https://www.acog.org/womens-health/faqs/how-to-tell-when-labor-begins

ACOG. (2020b, October). *Postpartum pain management.* ACOG. https://www.acog.org/womens-health/faqs/postpartum-pain-management

ACOG. (2021, May). *Bleeding during pregnancy.* ACOG. https://www.acog.org/womens-health/faqs/bleeding-during-pregnancy

Aggarwal, N. (2021, November 18). *Postpartum checkups: When they occur and what to expect.* Www.thebump.com. https://www.thebump.-com/a/postpartum-checkup

Alcohol and your pregnancy. (2022, August). National Institute on Alcohol Abuse and Alcoholism (NIAAA). https://www.niaaa.nih.gov/publications/brochures-and-fact-sheets/alcohol-and-your-pregnancy

Ali, U. A., & Norwitz, E. R. (2009). Vacuum-assisted vaginal delivery. *Reviews in Obstetrics and Gynecology, 2(1),* 5–17. https://www.ncbi.nlm.nih.-gov/pmc/articles/PMC2672989/#:~:text=Vacuum%2Dassisted%20vaginal%20deliveries%20can

American Cancer Society. (2023, February 1). *Benzene and cancer risk.* American Cancer Society. https://www.cancer.org/cancer/risk-prevention/chemicals/benzene.html

American College of Obstetricians and Gynecologists. (2020, April). *Physical activity and exercise during pregnancy and the postpartum period.* American College of Obstetricians and Gynecologists. https://www.acog.org/clinical/clinical-guidance/committee-opinion/articles/2020/04/physical-activity-and-exercise-during-pregnancy-and-the-postpartum-period

American Pregnancy Association. (n.d.-a). *Baby blues.* American Pregnancy Association. https://americanpregnancy.org/healthy-pregnancy/first-year-of-life/baby-blues/

American Pregnancy Association. (n.d.-b). *Baby development month by month.* American Pregnancy Association. https://americanpregnancy.org/healthy-pregnancy/week-by-week/baby-development-month-by-month/

American Pregnancy Association. (n.d.-c). *Breastfeeding vs bottle feeding.* American Pregnancy Association. https://americanpregnancy.org/healthy-pregnancy/breastfeeding/breastfeeding-vs-bottle-feeding-formula/

American Pregnancy Association. (n.d.-d). *Natural childbirth techniques.* American Pregnancy Association. https://americanpregnancy.org/healthy-pregnancy/labor-and-birth/natural-childbirth-techniques/

American Pregnancy Association. (n.d.-e). *Patterned breathing during labor.* American Pregnancy Association. https://americanpregnancy.org/healthy-pregnancy/labor-and-birth/patterned-breathing/

American Pregnancy Association. (n.d.-f). *Retained placenta.* American Pregnancy Association. https://americanpregnancy.org/healthy-pregnancy/labor-and-birth/retained-placenta/

Anderson, R., Rothwell, E., & Botkin, J. R. (2011). Newborn screening. *Annual Review of Nursing Research, 29,* 113–132. https://doi.org/10.1891/0739-6686.29.113

Ansong-Assoku, B., Ankola, P. A., Shah, S. D., & Adnan, M. (2023, February 20). *Neonatal jaundice.* National Library of Medicine. https://www. ncbi. nlm. nih. gov/ books/ NBK532930/

Artal-Mittelmark, R. (2022, September). *Stages of development of the fetus.* MSD Manuals. https://www.msdmanuals.com/home/women-s-health-issues/normal-pregnancy/stages-of-development-of-the-fetus

ASA. (2014, June 4). *Laboring under misconceptions: Epidural myths may keep women from reliable pain management.* American Society of Anesthesiologists. https://www.asahq.org/about-asa/newsroom/news-releases/2014/06/epidural-myth

Atkin, E. (n.d.). *Celeb mums who've had a water birth.* MadeForMums. https://www.madeformums.com/pregnancy/celebrity-mums-who-had-a-water-birth/

Balaram, K., & Marwaha, R. (2023, March 6). *Postpartum blues.* PubMed. https://www.ncbi.nlm.nih.gov/books/NBK554546/

Banoofatemeh, S., Oreyzi, H. R., & Bahadoran, P. (2017). *Effects of implementing the Alexander technique on enjoying the sense of motherhood in the postpartum period*. Iranian Journal of Nursing and Midwifery Research, 22(5), 392–397. https://doi.org/10.4103/ijnmr.IJNMR_26_16

Basevi, V., & Lavender, T. (2014). *Routine perineal shaving on admission in labour*. The Cochrane Database of Systematic Reviews, 2014(11). https://doi.org/10.1002/14651858.CD001236.pub2

Bellefonds, C. de. (2021, April 26). *How to recognize the symptoms of postpartum depression*. What to Expect. https://www.whattoexpect.com/first-year/postpartum-depression

Ben-Joseph, E. P. (2018, June). *Breastfeeding vs. formula feeding (for parents) - KidsHealth*. Kidshealth.org. https://kidshealth.org/en/parents/breast-bottle-feeding.html

Better Health Channel. (2017, April 27). *Pregnancy and exercise*. Victoria State Government. https://www.betterhealth.vic.gov-.au/health/healthyliving/pregnancy-and-exercise

Better Health Channel. (2022, April 19). *Ovulation*. Victoria State Government. https://www.betterhealth.vic.gov.au/health/condition-sandtreatments/ ovulation

Better Health Channel. (2022, June 9). *Pregnancy—medication, drugs and alcohol*. Victoria State Government. https://www.betterhealth.vic.gov-.au/health/healthyliving/pregnancy-medication-drugs-and-alcohol

Better Health Channel. (2022, July 9). *Ovulation*. Victoria State Government. https://www.betterhealth.vic.gov.au/health/conditionsandtreatments/ ovulation

Better Health Channel. (n.d.). *Alexander technique*. Victoria State Government. https://www.betterhealth.vic.gov.au/health/condition-sandtreatments/alexander-technique

Bible Gateway passage: Psalm 127:3 - New King James Version. (2015). Bible Gateway; BibleGateway. https://www.biblegateway.com/passage/? search=Psalm+127%3A3&version=NKJV

BMJ. (2020, August 24). *No safe level of caffeine consumption for pregnant women and would-be mothers*. BMJ. https://www.bmj.com/company/newsroom/no-safe-level-of-caffeine-consumption-for-pregnant-women-and-would-be-mothers/

Bradley, S. (2020, July 29). *6 months pregnant: Symptoms, belly, baby's development, more*. Healthline. https://www.healthline.com/health/pregnancy/6-months-pregnant#fetal-movement

The Bump. (2021, February 24). *How to deal with stress during pregnancy*.

The Bump. https://www.thebump.com/a/how-to-deal-with-stress-during-pregnancy

Buran, G., & Aksu, H. (2022). Effect of hypnobirthing training on fear, pain, satisfaction related to birth, and birth outcomes: a randomized controlled trial. *Clinical Nursing Research*, 31(5), 105477382110733. https://doi.org/10.1177/10547738211073394

Buser, G. L., Mató, S., Zhang, A. Y., Metcalf, B. J., Beall, B., & Thomas, A. R. (2017). Notes from the field: Late-onset infant group B streptococcus infection associated with maternal consumption of capsules containing dehydrated placenta. *MMWR. Morbidity and Mortality Weekly Report, 66*(25), 677–678. https://doi.org/10.15585/mmwr.mm6625a4

Calyx, L. (2018, January 13). *50+ motherhood quotes*. Pollen Nation. https://blog.serenataflowers.com/pollennation//motherhood-quotes/

Carlson, J. (2020, February 27). *8 dangers of smoking while pregnant*. Healthline. https://www.healthline.com/health/smoking-and-pregnancy

CDC. (2017, August 10). *Tdap (Pertussis) vaccine and pregnancy.* Centers for Disease Control and Prevention. https:// www. cdc. gov/vaccines/ pregnancy/ hcp-toolkit/ tdap-vaccine-pregnancy. html#:~:text=Protection% 20from% 20pertussis% 20vaccines% 20does

CDC. (2020, October 19). *Pregnancy.* Centers for Disease Control and Prevention. https://www.cdc.gov/marijuana/health-effects/pregnancy.html

CDC. (2021, July 22). *What to expect while breastfeeding*. Centers for Disease Control and Prevention. https://www.cdc.gov/nutrition/InfantandToddlerNutrition/breastfeeding/what-to-expect.html

CDCTobaccoFree. (2022, May 5). *Smoking, pregnancy, and babies*. Centers for Disease Control and Prevention. https://www.cdc.gov/tobacco/campaign/tips/diseases/pregnancy.html#:~:text=Smoking%20doubles%20your%20risk%20of

CDC. (2022a, May 22). *Depression among women*. Centers for Disease Control and Prevention. https://www.cdc.gov/reproductivehealth/depression/index.htm

CDC. (2022b, June 17). *Women need 400 mcg of folic acid every day*. Centers for Disease Control and Prevention. https://www.cdc.gov/ncbddd/folicacid/features/folic-acid.html

CDC. (2023a, January 11). Preconception health and health care is important for all. Centers for Disease Control and Prevention. https://www.cdc.-

gov/preconception/overview.html#:~:text=Preconception%20health%20-care%20is%20the

CDC. (2023c, February 15). *Planning for pregnancy.* Centers for Disease Control and Prevention. https://www.cdc.gov/preconception/planning.html

CDC. (2023c, April 10). *Medication and pregnancy.* Centers for Disease Control and Prevention. https://www.cdc.gov/pregnancy/meds/treating-fortwo/index.html

Chamberlain, G., & Steer, P. (1999). ABC of labour care: Unusual presentations and positions and multiple pregnancy. *BMJ*, 318(7192), 1192–1194. https://doi.org/10.1136/bmj.318.7192.1192

Choudhari, R. G., Tayade, S. A., Venurkar, S. V., & Deshpande, V. P. (2022). A review of episiotomy and modalities for relief of episiotomy pain. *Cureus*. https://doi.org/10.7759/cureus.31620

Cleveland Clinic. (2018, January 1). *Pregnancy diet: foods to eat while pregnant.* Cleveland Clinic. https://my.clevelandclinic.org/health/articles/12593-pregnancy-nutrition

Cleveland Clinic. (2019, November 18). *Placenta pills: Why some new moms take them—and what doctors say about the risks.* Health Essentials from Cleveland Clinic. https://health.clevelandclinic.org/placenta-pills-why-some-new-moms-take-them-and-what-doctors-say-about-the-risks/

Cleveland Clinic. (2021, November 17). *Vaginal bleeding during pregnancy: Causes & treatment.* Cleveland Clinic. https://my.clevelandclinic.org/health/symptoms/22044-bleeding-during-pregnancy

Cleveland Clinic. (2022a, October 3). *Clogged milk duct: Causes, symptoms & treatment*. Cleveland Clinic. https://my.clevelandclinic.org/health/diseases/24239-clogged-milk-duct

Cleveland Clinic. (2022b, January 17). *Jaundice in newborns: Symptoms, causes & treatment*. Cleveland Clinic. https://my.clevelandclinic.org/health/diseases/22263-jaundice-in-newborns

Cleveland Clinic. (2022c, January 25). *Fundal height: Measurement, what it means & accuracy.* Cleveland Clinic. https://my.clevelandclinic.org/health/diagnostics/22294-fundal-height#:~:text=be%20each%20week%3F-

Cleveland Clinic. (2022d, February 4). *Placenta: overview, anatomy, function & complications*. Cleveland Clinic. https://my.clevelandclinic.org/health/body/22337-placenta

Cleveland Clinic. (2022e, February 16). *Fetal alcohol syndrome.* Cleveland

Clinic. https://my.clevelandclinic.org/health/diseases/15677-fetal-alcohol-syndrome

Cleveland Clinic. (2022f, March 14). *Umbilical cord care & appearance.* Cleveland Clinic. https://my.clevelandclinic.org/health/treatments/11308-umbilical-cord-appearance-and-care

Cleveland Clinic. (2022g, April 1). *Stages of labor: What to expect during labor & delivery*. Cleveland Clinic. https://my.clevelandclinic.org/health/symptoms/22640-stages-of-labor

Cleveland Clinic. (2022h, April 1). *20 week ultrasound (anatomy Scan).* Cleveland Clinic. https://my.clevelandclinic.org/health/diagnostics/22644-20-week-ultrasound#:~:text=The%2020%2Dweek%20ultrasound%20scan

Cleveland Clinic. (2022j, May 26). *Vaginal delivery: What to expect, benefits & complications.* Cleveland Clinic. https://my.clevelandclinic.org/health/articles/23097-vaginal-delivery

Cleveland Clinic. (2022k, June 12). *Forceps delivery: What to expect, risks & recovery.* Cleveland Clinic. https://my.clevelandclinic.org/health/treatments/23260-forceps-delivery

Cleveland Clinic. (2022l, July 10). *Pregnancy: types of delivery*. Cleveland Clinic. https://my.clevelandclinic.org/health/articles/9675-pregnancy-types-of-delivery#:~:text=Types%20of%20Delivery-

Cleveland Clinic. (2022m, August 14). *C-section (cesarean section): Procedure, risks & recovery.* Cleveland Clinic. https://my.clevelandclinic.org/health/treatments/7246-cesarean-birth-c-section#:~:text=A%20C%2Dsection%20(or%20cesarean

Cleveland Clinic. (2022n, October 7). *Types of delivery for pregnancy.* Cleveland Clinic. https://my.clevelandclinic.org/health/articles/9675-pregnancy-types-of-delivery

Cleveland Clinic. (2022o, October 17). *Breast engorgement: Causes, complications & treatment*. Cleveland Clinic. https://my.clevelandclinic.org/health/symptoms/24306-breast-engorgement

Cleveland Clinic. (2022p, October 21). *Teratogens: effects, types, risks & prevention.* Cleveland Clinic. https://my.clevelandclinic.org/health/articles/24325-teratogens#:~:text=A%20teratogen%20is%20a%20substance

Cleveland Clinic. (2023a, January 16). *Labor induction*. Cleveland Clinic. https://my.clevelandclinic.org/health/treatments/17698-labor-induction

Cleveland Clinic. (2023b, February 6). *Mastitis: causes, symptoms, treatment*

& prevention. Cleveland Clinic. https://my.clevelandclinic.org/health/diseases/15613-mastitis

Cleveland Clinic. (2023c, March 3). *Fetal development*. Cleveland Clinic. https://my.clevelandclinic.org/health/articles/7247-fetal-development-stages-of-growth

Cleveland Clinic. (2023d, March 10). *Labor pain relief: Options & side effects*. Cleveland Clinic. https://my.clevelandclinic.org/health/articles/4450-labor-pain-relief

Cleveland Clinic. (2023e, June 7). *What to pack in your hospital bag: a checklist*. Cleveland Clinic. https://health.clevelandclinic.org/what-to-pack-in-hospital-bag/

Cleveland Clinic. (2023f, June 9). *Colic*. Cleveland Clinic. https://my.clevelandclinic.org/health/diseases/10823-colic#:~:text=Colic%20means%20your%20otherwise%20healthy

Cleveland Clinic. (2023g, June 20). *What is fetal biometry?* Cleveland Clinic. https://my.clevelandclinic.org/health/diagnostics/25087-fetal-biometry

Cleveland Clinic. (2023h, September 6). *Stillborn baby/stillbirth: causes & symptoms | Cleveland Clinic*. Cleveland Clinic. https://my.clevelandclinic.org/health/diseases/9685-stillbirth

Cline, E. (2022, December 5). *105 pregnancy quotes*. Baby Chick. https://www.baby-chick.com/pregnancy-quotes/

Comparing infant formulas with human milk. (n.d.). National Library of Medicine. https://www. ncbi. nlm. nih. gov/ books/ NBK215837/

Crenshaw, J. (2007). Care practice #6: No separation of mother and baby, with unlimited opportunities for breastfeeding. *Journal of Perinatal Education, 16*(3), 39–43. https://doi.org/10.1624/105812407x217147

Crider, C. (2021, May 25). *8 months pregnant: Symptoms, belly, baby size*. Healthline. https://www.healthline.com/health/pregnancy/8-months-pregnant

Cummings, H. W. (2023, June). *To shave or not to shave: An ob-gyn's guide to pubic hair care*. ACOG. https://www.acog.org/womens-health/experts-and-stories/the-latest/to-shave-or-not-to-shave-an-ob-gyns-guide-to-pubic-hair-care

Danielsson, K. (2021, September 13). *7 miscarriage False Alarms*. Verywell Family. https://www.verywellfamily.com/early-pregnancy-worries-2371547

Danielsson, K. (2022a, November 2). *What's a teratogen and how does it affect my pregnancy?* Verywell Family. https://www.verywellfamily.com/that-are-teratogens-2371658

Danielsson, K. (2022b, December 1). *Neural tube defects*. Verywellfamily. https://www.verywellfamily.com/neural-tube-defects-ntds-2371296

Darouich , A. A., Liehr, T., Weise, A., Schlembach, D., Schleußner, E., Kiehntopf, M., & Schreyer, I. (2015). Alpha-fetoprotein and its value for predicting pregnancy outcomes: a re-evaluation. *Journal of Prenatal Medicine*, 9(3-4). https://www.ncbi.nlm.nih.gov/pmc/articles/PMC4909107/

Desai, N. M., & Tsukerman, A. (2023, July 24). *Vaginal delivery*. PubMed. https://www.ncbi.nlm.nih.gov/books/NBK559197/

Desiraju, M. (2022, June). *Burping your baby (for parents)*. Kidshealth. https://kidshealth.org/en/parents/burping.html

Developing a birth plan. (2022, March 23). Victoria State Government. https://www.betterhealth.vic.gov.au/health/ServicesAndSupport/developing-a-birth-plan

Dugas, C., & Slane, V. H. (2022, June 27). *Miscarriage*. National Library of Medicine. https:// www. ncbi. nlm. nih. gov/ books/ NBK532992/

Edwards, A. (2019, April 12). *How to make 7 amazingly perfect pregnancy breakfast*. The Perfect Pregnancy Plan. https://theperfectpregnancyplan.-com/breastfast-ideas-pregnant-women/

11 Weeks pregnant—week-by-week guide. (n.d.). NHS. https://www.nhs.uk/start-for-life/pregnancy/week-by-week-guide-to-pregnancy/1st-trimester/week-11/

Embryonic & fetal development (p. 6). (2015). DHEC. https://scdhec.-gov/sites/default/files/Library/ML-017049.pdf

familydoctor.org Editorial Staff. (2023, May 1). *Tobacco, alcohol, and drugs during pregnancy*. Familydoctor.org. https://familydoctor.org/tobacco-alcohol-drugs-pregnancy/

Felton, A. (2022, August 20). *What to know about teratogens and birth defects*. WebMD. https://www.webmd.com/baby/what-to-know-about-teratogen-and-birth-defects

Fertility Center of Dallas. (n.d.). *7 tips to make your path to parenthood easier*. Fertility Center of Dallas. https://fertilitycenterofdallas.com/blog/7-tips-to-make-your-path-to-parenthood-easier/

Frothingham, S. (2018, July 24). *Lamaze breathing*. Healthline. https://www.healthline.com/health/lamaze-breathing#breathing-techniques

Garrard, C. (2020, December 2). *Celebrities who've had miscarriages and spoken out*. Everyday Health. https://www.everydayhealth.com/fertility/famous-women-miscarriages-spoken/

Gogol, F. (2023, June 19). *How to get a social security card for a newborn*. Stilt Blog. https://www.stilt.com/blog/2021/10/how-to-get-a-social-security-card-for-a-newborn/

Guarnotta, E. (2023, August 10). *Coping with stress during pregnancy: 10 ways to stay calm*. Choosing Therapy. https://www.choosingtherapy.com/stress-during-pregnancy/

Gupta, R. C. (2023, April). *Taking care of your mental health during pregnancy*. Kidshealth. https://kidshealth.org/en/parents/pregnant-mental-health.html

Gurevich, R. (2021, October 26). *What to know about the Bradley method of childbirth*. Verywell Family. https://www.verywellfamily.com/the-bradley-method-4586903

Gutzeit, O., LBotoxsxm.2019.10.005

Harnish, A. (2023, May 23). *How to change your baby's diaper*. What to Expect. https://www.whattoexpect.com/first-year/diapering/how-to-change-a-diaper/

Harris, N. (2023, July 2). *The best exercises to induce labor naturally*. Parents. https://www.parents.com/pregnancy/giving-birth/labor-and-delivery/7-exercises-to-induce-labor-you-can-do-at-home/#:~:text=Perform%20lunges

Harper, B. (2014). *Birth, bath, and beyond: The science and safety of water immersion during labor and birth*. The Journal of Perinatal Education, 23(3), 124–134. https://doi.org/10.1891/1058-1243.23.3.124

Hayes, E. H. (2016). Consumption of the placenta in the postpartum period. *Journal of Obstetric, Gynecologic & Neonatal Nursing, 45*(1), 78–89. https://doi.org/10.1016/j.jogn.2015.10.008

HealthHub. (2021, July 6). *What happens during your postnatal visit*. HealthHub. https://www. healthhub.sg/ live-healthy/ 1662/ what-happens- during- your- postnatal- visit

Healthline. (2023, July 28). *Pregnancy and teratogens: what you need to know*. Healthline. https://www.healthline.com/health/pregnancy/teratogens

Healthwise Staff. (2022, February 23). *Medicines during pregnancy*. Myhealth.Alberta. https://myhealth.alberta.ca/Health/Pages/conditions.aspx?hwid=uf9707

Henry Ford Health. (2019, June 11). *Baby blues vs postpartum depression: How to tell the difference.* Henry Ford Health. https://www.henryford.-com/blog/2019/06/baby-blues-vs-postpartum-depression

Henry Ford Health. (2021, January 11). *Beyond the baby blues: How to navigate your postpartum emotions.* Henry Ford Health. https://www.henryford.com/blog/2021/01/beyond-the-baby-blues-how-to-navigate-your-postpartum-emotions

Hidaka, R., & Callister, L. C. (2012). Giving birth with epidural analgesia: The experience of first-time mothers. *The Journal of Perinatal Education, 21*(1), 24–35. https://doi.org/10.1891/1058-1243.21.1.24

Higuera, V. (2016, December 20). *Recovery and care after delivery.* Healthline Media. https://www.healthline.com/health/postpartum-care#outlook

Horsager-Boehrer, R. (2015, January 6). *Planning a "gender-reveal" party? Some practical considerations.* UT Southwestern Medical Center. https://utswmed.org/medblog/gender-reveal/

Horsager-Boehrer, R. (2021, August 17). *1 in 10 dads experience postpartum depression, anxiety: How to spot the signs.* UT Southwestern Medical Center. https://utswmed.org/medblog/paternal-postpartum-depression/

Howell, C. J., Dean, T., Lucking, L., Dziedzic, K., Jones, P. W., & Johanson, R. B. (2002). Randomised study of long term outcome after epidural versus non-epidural analgesia during labour. *BMJ (Clinical Research Ed.)*, 325(7360), 357. https://www. ncbi. nlm. nih. gov/ pmc/ articles/ PMC117883/

HPHC. (n.d.). *Healthy parents healthy children.* Healthy Parents Healthy Children. https://www. healthyparentshealthychildren. ca/im-pregnant/ overview-of-pregnancy/ mental-health/#mental-health-changes

Jacobs, R. (2019, July 7). *Choosing where to give birth: Do you know all of your birth options?* Baby Chick. https://www.baby-chick.com/choosing-where-to-give-birth-do-you-know-all-of-your-birth-options/

Jin, J. (2022). Safety of Medications Used During Pregnancy. *JAMA*, 328(5), 486. https://doi.org/10.1001/jama.2022.8974

Kaur, A., & Kaur, A. (2011). *Transvaginal ultrasonography in first trimester of pregnancy and its comparison with transabdominal ultrasonography.* Journal of Pharmacy and Bioallied Sciences, 3(3), 329. https://doi.org/10.4103/0975-7406.84432

Konrad, G. (2007). First-trimester bleeding with falling hCG. *Canadian Family Physician*, 53(5), 831–832. https://www.ncbi.nlm.nih.-gov/pmc/articles/PMC1949168/

Kumar, K. (2021, September 16). *What are the different fetal positions?*

MedicineNet. https://www.medicinenet.com/what_are_the_different_fetal_positions/article.htm

Larson, J. (2020, August 27). *Can you get Botox while pregnant? Safety and Alternatives.* Healthline. https://www.healthline.com/health/pregnancy/botox-while-pregnant

LDH. (n.d.). *Stages of fetal development—third trimester.* LA Department of Health. https://ldh.la.gov/page/1059

Lee, W. A., Nelson, G., & Grogan, S. P. (2023, July 31). *Sonography 1st trimester assessment, protocols, and interpretation.* PubMed. https://www.ncbi.nlm.nih.gov/books/NBK573070/

Life in the womb. (n.d.). Indiana Right To Life. https://irtl.org/resources/life-in-the-womb/

Liles, M. (2023, May 18). *100 Pregnancy quotes for moms-to-be that describe what being pregnant is all about.* Parade: Entertainment, Recipes, Health, Life, Holidays. https://parade.com/971665/marynliles/pregnancy-quotes/

Lo, J. Y. (2022, April 19). *What moms should know about forceps and vacuum deliveries.* UT Southwestern Medical Center. https://utswmed.org/medblog/forceps-vacuum-delivery/

Longman, H. (2022, June 29). *How to get a social security card for a newborn.* BabyCenter. https://www.babycenter.com/family/money/social-security-numbers-and-why-your-baby-needs-one_1454647

Lothian, J. A. (2011). Lamaze breathing. *The Journal of Perinatal Education*, *20*(2), 118–120. https://doi.org/10.1891/1058-1243.20.2.118

Louisiana Department of Health. (n.d.). *Stages of fetal development—first trimester.* LA Dept. of Health. https://ldh.la.gov/page/986

Lumencandela. (n.d.). *Teratogens.* Lumencandela. https://courses.lumenlearning.com/suny-lifespandevelopment/chapter/teratogens/

M, K. (2023, July 14). *40 beautiful and inspirational pregnancy quotes and sayings.* MomJunction. https://www.momjunction.com/articles/beautiful-quotes-about-pregnancy_002953/

Ma, C. (2023, February 8). *10 safety guidelines that should be followed to welcome your newborn home.* Momcozy. https://momcozy.com/blogs/news/10-safety-guidelines-that-should-be-followed-to-welcome-your-newborn-home

Madden, K., Middleton, P., Cyna, A. M., Matthewson, M., & Jones, L. (2016). Hypnosis for pain management during labour and childbirth.

Cochrane Database of Systematic Reviews, 5. https://doi.org/10.1002/14651858.cd009356.pub3

Male reproductive system. (n.d.). Vecteezy. https://www.vecteezy.com/vector-art/418902-diagram-showing-male-reproductive-system

March of Dimes. (2019, February). *Safe sleep for your baby.* March of Dimes. https://www.marchofdimes.org/find-support/topics/parenthood/safe-sleep-your-baby

Marcin, A. (2017, May 1). *How long does sperm live outside the body?* Healthline. https://www.healthline.com/health/how-long-can-sperm-live-outside-the-body#frozen-sperm

Marcin, A. (2019, November 27). *Clogged milk duct: Symptoms, treatment, prevention, and more.* Healthline. https://www.healthline.-com/health/breastfeeding/clogged-milk-duct#causes

Matta, C. (2022, October 30). *Can I get Botox while pregnant?* Verywell Family. https://www.verywellfamily.com/can-i-get-botox-when-pregnant-5198014#:~:text=Risks%20of%20Using%20Botox%20While%20Pregnant

Mathew, P., & Bordoni, B. (2023, August 14). *Embryology, heart.* PubMed. https:// www. ncbi. nlm.nih. gov/ books/ NBK537313/ #:~:text= The% 20primitive% 20heart% 20tube% 20is

Mauldin, A. (n.d.). *Teratogen: what is it, examples, and more.* Osmosis. https://www.osmosis.org/answers/teratogen

Mayo Clinic. (2018, January 10). *Fetal alcohol syndrome—Symptoms and causes.* Mayo Clinic. https://www.mayoclinic.org/diseases-conditions/fetal-alcohol-syndrome/symptoms-causes/syc-20352901#:~:text=Fetal%20alcohol%20syndrome%20is%20a

Mayo Clinic. (2021, October 19). *Dilation and curettage (D&C).* Mayo Clinic. https://www.mayoclinic.org/tests-procedures/dilation-and-curettage/about/pac-20384910#:~:text=In%20a%20dilation%20and%20curettage

Mayo Clinic. (2022, December 6). *Kegel exercises: A how-to guide for women.* Mayo Clinic. https://www.mayoclinic.org/healthy-lifestyle/womens-health/in-depth/kegel-exercises/art-20045283

McKay, L. (2019, July 2). *What is the fertile window? | when am i fertile?* Natural Cycles. https://www.naturalcycles.com/cyclematters/what-is-the-fertile-window

MDH. (2023, April 4). Newborn screening information for providers: Blood spot screening Results. Minnesota Dept. of Health. https://www.health.s-tate.mn.us/people/newbornscreening/providers/bloodresults.html

MedicalNewsToday. (2022, June 28). *What to know about Apgar scores.* MedicalNewsToday. https://www.medicalnewstoday.com/articles/apgar-scores#apgar-score-test

MedlinePlus. (2021, July 13). *Fetal development: MedlinePlus Medical Encyclopedia.* Medlineplus.gov. https://medlineplus.gov/ency/article/002398.htm

MedlinePlus. (2022, April 19). *Episiotomy—aftercare.* MedlinePlus medical encyclopedia. https:// medlineplus.gov/ ency/ patientinstructions/ 000483.htm

Meixner, M. (2018, November 20). *Caffeine during pregnancy: how much is safe?* Healthline. https://www.healthline.com/nutrition/caffeine-during-pregnancy#safety

Milbrand, L. (2023, May 30). *Newborn baby bootcamp: Taking care of a newborn.* Parents. https://www.parents.com/baby/care/american-baby-how-tos/newborn-baby-boot-camp/

Miles, K. (2021, June 21). *10 ways to avoid gaining too much pregnancy weight.* BabyCenter. https://www.babycenter.com/pregnancy/health-and-safety/10-ways-to-avoid-gaining-too-much-pregnancy-weight_10396224

Molnar, C., & Gair, J. (2015). 13.2 *Development and organogenesis.* BCcampus. https://opentextbc.ca/biology/chapter/13-2-development-and-organogenesis/#:~:text=germ%20layers%20form.-

Mota-Rojas, D., Orihuela, A., Strappini, A., Villanueva-García, D., Napolitano, F., Mora-Medina, P., Barrios-García, H. B., Herrera, Y., Lavalle, E., & Martínez-Burnes, J. (2020). Consumption of maternal placenta in humans and nonhuman mammals: Beneficial and adverse effects. *Animals, 10*(12), 2398. https://doi.org/10.3390/ani10122398

Mustela. (n.d.). *7 months pregnant: symptoms, baby development, and tips.* Mustela USA. https://www.mustelausa.com/blogs/mustela-mag/7-months-pregnant#symptoms

Neilson, J. P. (1998). *Symphysis-fundal height measurement in pregnancy.* Cochrane Database of Systematic Reviews. https://doi.org/10.1002/14651858.cd000944

Neural tube defects (NTDs): What they are, causes & prevention. (2022, March 30). Cleveland Clinic. https://my.clevelandclinic.org/health/diseases/22656-neural-tube-defects-ntd#:~:text=Fetal%20(prenatal)%20ultrasound%3A%20An

NHS. (2018, December 13). *Sex and contraception after birth.* NHS. https://www.nhs.uk/conditions/baby/support-and-services/sex-and-contraception-after-birth/

NHS. (2020a, February 14). *Vitamins, minerals and supplements in pregnancy*. NHS. https://www.nhs.uk/pregnancy/keeping-well/vitamins-supplements-and-nutrition/

NHS. (2020b, September 29). *Postpartum psychosis*. NHS. https://www.nhs.uk/mental-health/conditions/post-partum-psychosis/

NHS. (2020c, November 30). *Signs that labour has begun*. NHS. https://www.nhs.uk/pregnancy/labour-and-birth/signs-of-labour/signs-that-labour-has-begun/

NHS. (2021a, February 1). *Tiredness and sleep problems*. NHS. https://www.nhs.uk/pregnancy/related-conditions/common-symptoms/tiredness/

NHS. (2021b, February 19). *Mental health problems and pregnancy*. NHS. https://www.nhs.uk/pregnancy/keeping-well/mental-health/

NHS. (2021c, March 16). *Stillbirth—causes*. NHS. https://www.nhs.uk/conditions/stillbirth/causes/

NHS. (2021d, April 14). *How to make a birth plan*. NHS. https://www.nhs.uk/pregnancy/labour-and-birth/preparing-for-the-birth/how-to-make-a-birth-plan/

NHS. (2022a, February 3). *Newborn jaundice*. NHS. https://www.nhs.uk/conditions/Jaundice-newborn/

NHS. (2022b, August 22). *What complications can affect the placenta?* NHS. https://www.nhs.uk/pregnancy/labour-and-birth/what-happens/placenta-complications/

NHS. (2022c, June 27). *Circumcision in boys*. NHS. https://www.nhs.uk/conditions/circumcision-in-boys/

NHS. (2022d, October 4). *Washing and bathing your baby*. NHS. https://www.nhs.uk/conditions/baby/caring-for-a-newborn/washing-and-bathing-your-baby/

NHS. (2022e, November 28). *Your 6-week postnatal check*. NHS. https://www.nhs.uk/conditions/baby/support-and-services/your-6-week-postnatal-check/

NHS. (2023a, January 4). *Overview—Caesarean section*. NHS. https://www.nhs.uk/conditions/caesarean-section/

NHS. (2023b, March 13). *Pain relief in labour*. NHS. https://www.nhs.uk/pregnancy/labour-and-birth/what-happens/pain-relief-in-labour/

NHS. (2023c, March 14). *Forceps or vacuum delivery*. NHS.

https://www.nhs.uk/pregnancy/labour-and-birth/what-happens/forceps-or-vacuum-delivery/

NHS. (2023d, March 15). *Exercise in pregnancy.* NHS. https://www.nhs.uk/pregnancy/keeping-well/exercise/

NHS. (2023e, March 17). *Overview—mastitis.* NHS. https://www.nhs.uk/conditions/mastitis/

NIAAA. (2022, August). *Alcohol and your pregnancy.* National institute on alcohol abuse and alcoholism (NIAAA). https://www.niaaa.nih.gov/publications/brochures-and-fact-sheets/alcohol-and-your-pregnancy#:~:text=A%20developing%20baby%20is%20exposed

NIAAA. (2023, August). *Understanding fetal alcohol spectrum disorders.* National institute on alcohol abuse and alcoholism (NIAAA). https://www.niaaa.nih.gov/publications/brochures-and-fact-sheets/understanding-fetal-alcohol-spectrum-disorders

NIH. (2020, April). *Substance use while pregnant and breastfeeding.* National Institute on Drug Abuse. https://nida.nih.gov/publications/research-reports/substance-use-in-women/substance-use-while-pregnant-breast-feeding#:~:text=NAS%20occurs%20when%20heroin%20passes

NIH. (2020, October 22). *Glucose tolerance tests: What exactly do they involve?* National Library of Medicine. https:// www. ncbi. nlm. nih. gov/ books/ NBK279331/#:~:text=Glucose%20challenge%20test

NIH. (n.d.). *Teratogens/prenatal substance abuse.* National Library of Medicine. https://www. ncbi. nlm. nih. gov/ books/ NBK132140/

Oberg, E. (2022, April 15). *Childbirth types: Natural childbirth, water birth, home birth.* MedicineNet. https://www.medicinenet.com/7_childbirth_and_delivery_methods/article.htm

Osterman, M., & Martin, J. (2011). Epidural and spinal anesthesia use during labor: 27-state reporting area, 2008. *National Vital Statistics Reports*, 59(5). https://www.cdc.gov/nchs/data/nvsr/nvsr59/nvsr59_05.pdf

Overett, S. (2023, September 14). *The ultimate postpartum checklist of post-birth essentials.* Kin Fertility. https://kinfertility.com.au/blog/postpartum-checklist

Parents. (2023, August 10). *The best pelvic floor exercises during pregnancy.* Parents. https://www.parents.com/pregnancy/my-body/fitness/the-best-pelvic-floor-exercises-during-pregnancy/

Penn Medicine. (n.d.). *How to reduce stress during pregnancy.* Lancaster General Health. https://www.lancastergeneralhealth.org/health-hub-home/motherhood/your-pregnancy/how-to-reduce-stress-during-pregnancy

Perlman, N. C., & Carusi, D. A. (2019). Retained placenta after vaginal delivery: risk factors and management. *International Journal of Women's Health, Volume 11*(11), 527–534. https://doi.org/10.2147/ijwh.s218933

Petruska, Dr. S. E. (2022, February). *Making sense of childbirth pain relief options.* ACOG. https://www.acog.org/womens-health/experts-and-stories/the-latest/making-sense-of-childbirth-pain-relief-options

Pietrangelo, A. (2022, March 31). *Postpartum depression: Symptoms, treatment, causes & more.* Healthline. https://www.healthline.com/health/depression/postpartum-depression#causes-and-risk-factors

Preconception care: A guide for optimizing outcomes. (2021, February 22). New York State. https://www.health.ny.gov/publications/2026/

Pregnancy and birth: Epidurals and painkillers for labor pain relief. (2018, March 22). National Library of Medicine. https://www. ncbi.nlm. nih. gov/ books/ NBK279567/

Ramos, D. (2022, February). *What to expect at a postpartum checkup—and why the visit matters.* ACOG. https://www.acog.org/womens-health/experts-and-stories/the-latest/what-to-expect-at-a-postpartum-checkup-and-why-the-visit-matters

Radner, G. (n.d.). *Gilda Radner quote.* A-Z Quotes. https://www.azquotes.-com/quote/540709

Radzyminski, S., & Callister, L. C. (2016). Mother's beliefs, attitudes, and decision making related to infant feeding choices. *The Journal of Perinatal Education, 25*(1), 18–28. https://doi.org/10.1891/1058-1243.25.1.18

Raines, D. A., & Cooper, D. B. (2023, August 8). *Braxton Hicks contractions.* National Library of Medicine. https://www. ncbi. nlm. nih. gov/ books/ NBK470546/

Rawlins, A. (2016, August 23). *5 exercises and techniques to train for childbirth | Your pregnancy matters.* UT Southwestern Medical Center. https://utswmed.org/medblog/prepare-body-labor-delivery/

Raza, S. K., & Raza, S. (2023, June 26). *Postpartum psychosis.* PubMed. https:// www. ncbi.nlm.nih. gov/books/ NBK544304/ #:~:text=Postpartum% 20psychosis% 20is% 20the% 20severest

Rehman, B., & Muzio, M. R. (2023, May 1). *Embryology, week 2-3.* PubMed. https://www.ncbi.nlm.nih.gov/books/NBK546679/

Roberts, K. (2009, September 1). *Positive relationships: early learning—*

homing in. Nursery World. https://www.nurseryworld.co.uk/features/article/positive-relationships-early-learning-homing-in

Rockliffe, Dr. L. (2023, March 10). *The importance of social support in pregnancy and ways to connect with others.* Tommy's. https://www.tommys.org/pregnancy-information/pregnancy-news-blogs/pregnancy-news-blogs-being-pregnant/importance-social-support

Saha, R. (2023, August 17). *Top 15 healthy recipes for pregnant women*. MomJunction. https://www.momjunction.com/articles/healthy-recipes-for-pregnant-women_00347470/

Santilli, M. (2023, August 14). *What is water birthing? Everything you need to know*. Forbes Health. https://www.forbes.com/health/womens-health/pregnancy/guide-to-water-birthing/

Shahna. (2020, March 24). *5 healthy breakfast ideas for pregnancy*. Mum's Grapevine. https://mumsgrapevine.com.au/2020/03/breakfast-ideas-morning-sickness/

Shaw, A. (2022a, July 20). *Healthy and delicious first trimester recipes*. Baby Chick. https://www.baby-chick.com/healthy-delicious-first-trimester-recipes/

Shaw, A. (2022b, July 20). *Healthy and nutritious second trimester recipe*s. Baby Chick. https://www.baby-chick.com/healthy-and-nutritious-second-trimester-recipes/

Shaw, A. (2022c, July 20). *Healthy and high energy third trimester recipe*s. Baby Chick. https://www.baby-chick.com/healthy-and-high-energy-third-trimester-recipes/

Shojaei, B., Loripoor, M., Sheikhfathollahi, M., & Aminzadeh, F. (2021). The effect of walking during late pregnancy on the outcomes of labor and delivery: A randomized clinical trial. *Journal of Education and Health Promotion*, 10, 277. https://doi.org/10.4103/jehp.jehp_1437_20

Simpson, E., Carstensen, J., & Murphy, P. (2014). Neonatal circumcision: New recommendations & implications for practice. *Missouri Medicine, 111*(3), 222–230. https://www.ncbi.nlm.nih.gov/pmc/articles/PMC6179567/

Sivalingam, V. N., Duncan, W. C., Kirk, E., Shephard, L. A., & Horne, A. W. (2011). *Diagnosis and management of ectopic pregnancy*. Journal of Family Planning and Reproductive Health Care, 37(4), 231–240. https://doi.org/10.1136/jfprhc-2011-0073

Smith-Garcia, D. (2020, October 30). *The Bradley Method: What it is and how it works*. Healthline. https://www.healthline.com/health/pregnancy/bradley-method#pros

Sorgen, C. (2003, May 19). *Less stress during pregnancy for healthier mom, baby*. WebMD. https://www.webmd.com/parenting/features/less-stress-for-healthier-mom-baby

Souza, K. (2022, September 23). *Comforting postpartum depression quotes for 2022*. Choosing Therapy. https://www.choosingtherapy.com/postpartum-depression-quotes/

Sung, S., & Mahdy, H. (2023, July 9). *Cesarean section*. National Library of Medicine. https:// www. ncbi. nlm. nih. gov/ books/ NBK546707/

Tabin, E. (2023, June 8). *Here's why you shouldn't get Botox while pregnant—and what to try instead*. InStyle. https://www.instyle.com/botox-while-pregnant-7509708

Taylor, M. (2022b, March 23). *Are placenta pills safe?* What to Expect. https://www.whattoexpect.com/first-year/postpartum-health-and-care/placenta-encapsulation/

Terreri, C. (2016, December 22). *Different birth plans for different birth places*. Lamaze International. https://www.lamaze.org/Giving-Birth-with-Confidence/GBWC-Post/different-birth-plans-for-different-birth-places

13 inspiring quotes on giving birth. (2022, April 6). All Things Childcare. https://allthingschildcare.com/quotes-on-giving-birth/

Theo, L. O., & Drake, E. (2017). Rooming-In: Creating a better experience. *The Journal of Perinatal Education, 26*(2), 79–84. https://doi.org/10.1891/1058-1243.26.2.79

Tonismae, T., Canela, C. D., & Gossman, W. (2023, July 29). *Vacuum extraction*. PubMed. https://www.ncbi.nlm.nih.gov/books/NBK459234/

Trifu, S., Vladuti, A., & Popescu, A. (2019). Neuroendocrine aspects of pregnancy and postpartum depression. *Acta Endocrinologica (Bucharest), 15*(3), 410–415. https://doi.org/10.4183/aeb.2019.410

UnityPoint Health. (n.d.). *Male postpartum depression*. UnityPoint Health. https://www.unitypoint.org/news-and-articles/male-postpartum-depression--unitypoint-health

Valeii, K. (2021, April 23). *What is a teratogen?* Verywell Health. https://www.verywellhealth.com/teratogens-5118058

WebMD. (2022, November 30). *What is toxoplasmosis?* WebMD. https://www.webmd.com/baby/toxoplasmosis

Weiss, R. E. (2021, November 18). *What to know about your baby's position during labor and birth*. Verywell Family. https://www.verywellfamily.-

com/fetal-positions-for-labor-and-birth-2759020

Westmead Fertility Center. (2018, October 31). *How healthy lifestyle choices can improve your fertility.* Westmead Fertility Centre. https://www.westmeadfertilitycentre.com.au/how-healthy-lifestyle-choices-can-improve-your-fertility/

World Health Organization. (2013). *Postnatal care of the mother and newborn.* National Library of Medicine. https://www. ncbi. nlm. nih. gov/ books/ NBK304191/

Yekefallah, L., Namdar, P., Dehghankar, L., Golestaneh, F., Taheri, S., & Mohammadkhaniha, F. (2021). The effect of yoga on the delivery and neonatal outcomes in nulliparous pregnant women in Iran: A clinical trial study. *BMC Pregnancy and Childbirth*, 21(1). https://doi.org/10.1186/s12884-021-03794-6

Image References

Balielo Jr, V. (2014). *Doctor holding baby* [Image]. Pexels. https://www.pexels.com/photo/doctor-holding-baby-3376788/

Drp8. (n.d.). *Vector—cervical effacement and dilatation during labor* [Image]. Shutterstock. https://www.shutterstock.com/image-vector/vector-cervical-effacement-dilatation-during-labor-1574027293

Graphics RF. (n.d.). *Female reproductive system* [Image]. Vecteezy. https://www.vecteezy.com/vector-art/296631-diagram-showing-female-reproductive-system

Graphics RF. (n.d.). *Male reproductive system* [Image]. Vecteezy. https://www.vecteezy.com/vector-art/418902-diagram-showing-male-reproductive-system

Graphics RF. (n.d.). *Stages human embryonic development* [Image]. Vecteezy. https://www.vecteezy.com/vector-art/1437095-stages-human-embryonic-development

Lazebnaya, J. (2021). *Set of different pregnant women, dress, hijab, underwear. African american, arab woman, caucasian. Young beautiful multi-ethnic mothers of different nationalities. Diversity, multiethnic society* [Image]. iStock. https://www.istockphoto.com/vector/set-of-different-pregnant-women-dress-hijab-underwear-african-american-arab-woman-gm1301581571-393582584?phrase=beautiful+pregnant+woman+veiled

Martmoh, C. (n.d.). *The sperm is directed towards the egg. To do human mating. A pre-fertilization model between an egg and a sperm* [Image].

Vecteezy. https://www.vecteezy.com/photo/6660594-the-sperm-is-directed-towards-the-egg-to-do-human-mating-a-pre-fertilization-model-between-an-egg-and-a-sperm-3d-rendering

Ngamnithiporn, N. (n.d.). *Baked chicken breast stuffed with cheese and spinach* [Image]. Vecteezy. https://www.vecteezy.com/photo/2839103-baked-chicken-breast-stuffed-with-cheese-and-spinach

OpenClipart-Vectors. (2017). *Baby cartoon character* [Image]. Pixabay. https://pixabay.com/vectors/baby-cartoon-character-cigarette-2022446/

pamujiwish. (n.d.). *Cute baby vector flat illustration design* [Image]. Vecteezy. https://www.vecteezy.com/vector-art/21683683-cute-baby-vector-flat-illustration-design

Patapova, V. (n.d.). *Pregnant woman doing yoga, 8 exercises for health and relaxation* [Image]. Vecteezy. https://www.vecteezy.com/vector-art/15740343-pregnant-woman-doing-yoga-8-exercises-for-health-and-relaxation

RDNE Stock project. (2020). *Pregnancy test inside a gift box* [Image]. Pexels. https://www.pexels.com/photo/pregnancy-test-inside-a-gift-box-6148902/

Reche, D. (2016). *Photo of pregnant woman* [Image]. Pexels. https://www.pexels.com/photo/photo-of-pregnant-woman-1556652/

Robuart. (n.d.). *Birth active positions, information pregnant women. Supported squats, on fitball, standing on all fours, kneeling leaning prop in hospital water genera. Childbirth labor positions and postures at home* [Image]. Shutterstock. https://www.shutterstock.com/image-vector/birth-active-positions-information-pregnant-women-1478736860

Shumikhina, I. (n.d.). *A woman experiences side effects of pregnancy. Vector illustration of diseases during pregnancy* [Image]. Shutterstock. https://www.shutterstock.com/image-vector/woman-experiences-side-effects-pregnancy-vector-1313672906

Style graphic. (n.d.). *A delicious chicken soup food with vegetables in a bowl* [Image]. Vecteezy. https://www.vecteezy.com/photo/26585822-a-delicious-chicken-soup-food-with-vegetables-in-a-bowl-winter-food-and-high-protein-soup-meal-concept-by-ai-generated

Suwin. (n.d.). *Female reproductive system* [Image]. Shutterstock. https://www.shutterstock.com/image-illustration/female-reproductive-system-image-diagram-243154639

www.ingramcontent.com/pod-product-compliance
Lightning Source LLC
LaVergne TN
LVHW010320220926
848484LV00004BB/805